REGGIE

Making the Message Simple

Joseph B. Strauss, D.C., F.C.S.C.

Chiropractic Outside the Box
P.O. Box 142
Wernersville, PA 19565

For information on other materials available from COTB,
call 610-693-4039
or visit www.ChiropracticOutsidetheBox.com

To Reggie Gold
chiropractor, philosopher, teacher,
mentor, motivator, and friend

Author's Note

As one interested in the philosophy and the history of the chiropractic profession, particularly that of straight chiropractic, I have been keenly interested in writing this book. It is, hopefully, a chronicle of the recent history of straight chiropractic and the man most closely associated with it.

Some people will be disappointed that this is not a "tell-all" book. This book, like all my other books, is about chiropractic. It happens that Reggie Gold's life is inextricably woven into the profession. I have tried to be as objective as possible in giving a picture of the man as he relates to the profession and how his personality has impacted on chiropractic. I do confess that this book is also a tribute to Reggie Gold. As a nineteen-year old, first-semester chiropractic student I learned my chiropractic from Reggie. I have continued to learn from him for the last thirty-two years and I owe almost all my understanding of our chiropractic philosophy to him. This book, then, is also a way of saying thank you for an exciting and rewarding thirty-two years of learning and growing in the chiropractic philosophy. It is my hope that the reader will get a glimpse of what Reggie has meant to me and countless other chiropractors over the years and more importantly, what he has meant to chiropractic.

Acknowledgments

This book contains more acknowledgments than any other book I have written, which means that I have had more assistance in writing it than any other. First and foremost, thanks go to Reggie, who spent hours with me in his study as I poked and prodded into his personal life, his past and the deep recesses of his mind. He was extremely gracious and patient with me and my attempts at being an interviewer. After almost a year of periodic interviews, approximately every other month, I then began to make phone calls asking him a question or two to fill in some of the details. I appreciate his time and perseverance. I hope he finds this book worth his effort.

I also owe thanks to Irene Gold for her time in sharing insights into Reggie, the person. Dr. Dick Plummer of Inman, South Carolina spent a few hours with me, allowing me to grill him about Reggie. His information was invaluable. A number of the photographs, particularly the PACE (Patient Association for Chiropractic Education) photos came from his scrapbook. Dick also read the draft and offered valuable suggestions. Bryan Amaral, who as a non-chiropractic personal friend of Reggie's, gave me a unique look at Reggie. Dr. Tom Gregory gave me almost all of the information concerning Spinology, besides Reggie, including tapes, photographs, and school catalogs. Glenn Allen also was a help with the Spinology chapter. Rob Sinnott from Illinois was a lifesaver in acquiring a needed photograph. Special thanks also to Tom Murphy for providing us with the 1957 Palmer College Yearbook.

Thom Gelardi and Sherman College are owed special mention. Thom and the school have provided the friendship and environment for Reggie to accomplish much of what is contained in this book. Further, they have provided volumes of information and photos that aided my writing.

Joe Donoffio gave me insights and was gracious enough to read my draft. There are not too many people in chiropractic who go as far back with Reggie as Joe D. There were dozens of people who wrote letters, talked to me on the phone, and generally helped me put the information together to write this book. To each of you, my gratitude.

My faithful staff as always made barely readable handwritten notes into what you are about to read. Stacy Wilson and Kim Maddocks typed the original manuscript into the computer. My wife, Iris, edited and proof read it as she has my other books. Tracy Higley, my daughter, has done the layout and the difficult job of getting the photographs, some very old and some of very poor quality into the computer and ready for publication.

Last, but far from least is my associate, Dr. Judy Nutz Campanale. Judy has labored on every one of my books, since 1991. She spends countless hours editing each book. Any improvement of my writing over the years is largely due to her. Her contribution to *this* book is special, however. In May of 1995 I mentioned to her that one day I would like to write Reggie's biography. She convinced me to start it immediately, and so began the project that resulted in what is before you today. Thank you, Judy.

Table of Contents

Introduction

It has been said that history is really a chronicle of people's lives. To truly understand history, you must know the people who have lived it and made it. This is no more evident anywhere than in the history of chiropractic. The lives of D.D. and B.J. Palmer are the first half of our profession's history. They WERE chiropractic. Since B.J.'s passing there has been no personality whose fortunes mirror the development of the profession. That is not to suggest that there have not been a number of prominent individuals who have contributed to the development of the profession. But no single individual is identified with chiropractic as were the Founder and Developer for more than fifty years.

The same cannot be said about the segment of the chiropractic profession that identifies itself as straight. The name Reggie is almost synonymous with straight chiropractic. He has been its chief spokesman and proponent for almost thirty years. To students, chiropractors, lay people and the health field community he has shown many sides, that of philosopher, teacher, leader, educator and motivator to name a few. His ability to articulate straight chiropractic is admired throughout the profession (begrudgingly admired by some). His generosity to chiropractic, in general, and Sherman College of Straight Chiropractic, in particular, is well known. What is not so well known is the personal, individual impact he has had on thousands of lives through the simple but eloquent articulation of the straight chiropractic philosophy. A few excerpts from letters of those who have chosen to acknowledge the profound effect he has had on their lives are included here.

Reggie,

I am grateful for your kindness, your endless generosity, the respectful and thoughtful way you answered my questions over the years and helped me to find my own answers.

P.

Reggie,

Well, Reggie, I gave my first C-5 supine adjustment yesterday. It was very exciting. I am so excited about my chiropractic future I can hardly sleep at night. Thank you Reggie, for all you are.

T.

Dear Reggie,

Words cannot express the impact your teaching and shared wisdom have made on us. And this page is too small to attempt it.

B., C. and J.

Dear Reggie,

I first heard you several years ago, but I didn't buy all of what you were presenting. This time it got through. It is the first time I have really been excited about practice.

B.

Hi Reg,

...What I have learned about chiropractic all came from you. I would never have gone as far as I have if not for the enthusiasm created by you and your love of chiropractic principle.

T.

Dear Reggie,

...I see chiropractic with new eyes, and have a deeper respect since listening to your seminar.

J.

Dear Reg,

If there is one person who is responsible more than any other for saving this profession, it is you. Your educating so many, your inspiring those capable of being inspired and your example of service, generosity and love had a truly significant effect on TIC still being here.

T.

Dear Reggie,

Without your seminar I may never have found myself and chiropractic.

N.

Reg,

...My eyes were opened to the art and philosophy of chiropractic after listening, what a "revelation" to me.

B.

Dear Reggie,

I am truly a better person as a result of our relationship and will always use tenacious fortitude to uphold the principles of Straight Chiropractic, thus ensuring its acceptance and understanding.

L.

Reggie,

Thousands of D.C.s help thousands more patients because of you. My admiration and respect are yours.

L.

Reggie,

You'll never know how much you've changed my aspects on chiropractic for the better. You are and will always be to me, the greatest communicator of chiropractic there is...

D.

Dear Reg,

Your love for chiropractic and humanity is an inspiration to me and to the profession.

G.

Dear Reggie,

Thank you for sharing with me your thoughts and feelings so that I may better see the truth. After feeling confused about chiropractic since my "education" has begun, I feel that now I am starting to see true chiropractic.

Warmest Regards,
M.

Dear Reggie,

I was deeply moved by your presentation during the weekend. For the first time, the philosophy of chiropractic was presented to me in a manner which rang true.

With love and appreciation,
L.

Dear Reggie,

They [the tapes] have helped us already to reposition our practice to a more wellness-oriented one (which is what we've wanted to do all along and haven't quite known how) and have let us resolve several conflicts of principles, and consequently, we've let go of a lot of unneeded stress.

T.

Dear Reggie,

Thank you for being all that you are and reminding me of all that I may yet become.

In health,
D.

Reggie,

In all the seminars, in all the towns, in all the world you had to pick mine to walk into. Lucky us. Thank you. You'll never know how far reaching...

D.

Dear Reggie,

My wife and I just finished listening to the entire series of tapes tonight. This culminates the most exciting week in practice I have had in over two years. You and your tapes have given me a real basis for my chiropractic existence and a philosophy that we didn't get in practice. After eight years in practice, I now know the answer to several questions and doubts I had about Chiropractic and even myself. For that I owe you a great deal. Thank you.

K.

Dear Reggie,

You have touched my life and therefore my world like few people have done in the past. I thank you so much for myself and for the hundreds of families that will have the privilege to be under chiropractic care for a lifetime.

Love and Respect
C.

Dear Reggie,

Your talk was truly inspiring and motivating in re-discovering your purposes and the true meaning of chiropractic.

J.

Hello Reggie,

Thank you for speaking at ...I'm afraid you hit me right between the eyes. I have allowed the dimmer switch of negative feedback to dampen my vision and mission. Thank you for the wake-up call.

J.

Dear Reggie,

Because of what you said this past Thursday, you have given me back my vision which I have lost during eleven years in the alligator pit...

Most sincerely,
R.

Dear Reggie,

As our philosophy teacher, you were responsible for the opening of our understanding, which directly affected the quality and the richness of our lives.

M.

Dear Reggie,

You have saved me from a musculoskeletal career of patching up Sciatica as taught at...

Thanks again,
P.

Below are excerpts from two of the many letters sent to me when it was made known that I was writing Reggie's biography.

Dear Dr. Strauss,

It's not often I meet someone that touches my life in a special way as to have made such an impact on it. When I first heard Reggie speak early on in chiropractic college, I said to myself, "Yes! Finally someone is telling the simple truth." Reggie's passion, love, uniqueness, and zest for life and the truth has made a big imprint on my life. As I go out and begin my journey as a chiropractor, I am honored to have been touched by such a beautiful human being.

D.

Dear Dr. Strauss,

...Through Reggie I have learned how to think logically for myself instead of reacting fearfully. This has given me the opportunity to communicate chiropractic eloquently in a way everyone can understand the vital role we (chiropractic) play in humanity. Most importantly the understanding of chiropractic philosophy learned through Reggie has created the strong foundation from which to grow, defend and communicate our vision to the masses...

N.

The human body appears at first glance to be a simple mechanism. Two eyes, a nose, a mouth, arms and legs. However, the more you investigate it the more complex and marvelous it becomes. The complexity of a simple movement like flexing the arm is a beautiful demonstration of coordination, order and organization. The intricacies of the human eye and the function of sight is awe-inspiring. The closer your investigation, the more complicated it becomes. Eventually, we realize that the complexity of the human cell is more that we can understand. The attempts at an explanation of it have filled volumes and have yet to scratch the surface of its complexity.

The chiropractic philosophy at first appears to be very simple, in fact, to many it seems to be too simple. But the more you understand and develop the chiropractic philosophy, the more complex, the more interesting and exciting its principles and ramifications become. Most importantly, the more you understand it, the more it is applicable to life and allows for a fuller understanding and expression of this complex phenomena that we call the human experience. Eventually it moves into metaphysical areas that we cannot truly comprehend. We have barely begun to understand the ramifications of our philosophy.

Just as with the human body and the chiropractic philosophy, Reggie, the man, is complex upon investigation. His message, from which he rarely deviates, is clear and fundamental, and yet we will probably never fully understand the man, his desires in life, his ideas, feelings, goals. We do know that he is distinctive in that his life revolves around one thing - chiropractic. To understand Reggie and his life is to understand the development of straight chiropractic for at least as long as he has been associated with it. What is the man Reggie Gold like, what drives him? Reggie is chiropractic and it is what drives him, at least that is what is apparent on the surface. Like the human body and the philosophy there are parts of Reggie as a human being that no one can understand, perhaps not even Reggie. The same could be said of all of us. Perhaps by learning of his life, we can learn more of our profession, our philosophy and even ourselves.

CHAPTER 1

London, England to Davenport, Iowa

Birth to 1957

The clipped English accent belies the fact that Reggie Gold was born in the East London borough of Bow, making him about as cockney as one can be. Like the Eliza Doolittle character in Lemer and Loewe's "My Fair Lady," he overcame the distinctive cockney accent. Reggie's life is marked by overcoming obstacles, both personally and professionally, and a burning desire to succeed in the face of adversity. So it is no surprise that he should overcome the cockney intonation, retaining just enough of his English accent to endear himself to any listener and become, in the opinion of many, the most articulate speaker in the chiropractic profession.

His early childhood growing up in London was markedly unexceptional. He lived in pre-war London with two brothers, a sister and his mother and father. His earliest recollection of home was, in his words, "a slum." Most large cities had ghettos where similar ethnic groups resided. Reggie's father was a candy maker and as the children grew older he received more income for his work and they were able to afford to move to better housing. Like many people growing up in a similar environment, Reggie was motivated by his humble beginnings to get ahead. His sister Lee, who was the oldest sibling, was five and a half years older than Reggie. At the time of this writing she is living in Tucson, Arizona. The next oldest was Jack who is now deceased. Jack was four years older than Reggie. The youngest, Martin, was five years younger than

Reggie. The difference in years between Reggie and his siblings caused him as a young boy to be a loner, although the family as a whole was very close-knit in the early years. They were typical of a Jewish-European family. Reg's first recollection of employment was as a sweeper in a pawn shop at age eleven. He had dropped out of school at that age with the equivalent of a sixth-grade education, a not uncommon occurrence for a young boy at the time. With the impending war (England entered the war in 1939, two years before the United States), an education was not a priority for an eleven-year old growing up in East London. Priority was helping the family put food on the table. The Great Depression that preceded World War II was not only confined to the United States, so Reggie, like his older sister and brother, went to work. Although not pursuing formal education, he was still learning. He continues to be an avid reader and student of life. An education in the things of the world was forced upon young Reggie. There appears to be no single childhood incident or experience that created the environment or the driving force that produced the character and the qualities that make up Reggie Gold, the chiropractor. There were many events that influenced Reg Gold, the man, from his poverty, his working at an early age to the death of his younger brother who took his own life at the age of 19. There was nothing in his childhood that pointed him toward or away from the health field. Matters of health were simply not important in England at the time, especially in the less affluent areas. People did not run to the doctor except for serious conditions. Other than childhood diseases and an appendectomy, Reggie was not a sickly child. His first real experience with what might be described as the shortcoming of medicine was in his late teens while on leave from the army. He developed the symptoms of hepatitis. He recognized it because fifty other soldiers in camp had been treated for it. He saw a local medical doctor who examined him and diagnosed appendicitis. Reg knew it was hepatitis because the symptoms were the same as the other soldiers and because he had already had his appendix removed! But that experience did not turn him off to medicine. Like most people, he merely wrote it off as one incompetent medical doctor.

While his parents "were not terribly religious," in his opinion, they were insistent that he be raised in the Jewish faith. Perhaps their thinking was that he could neither accept nor reject the faith unless he was familiar with it. While Judaism had little effect on his life, his race as a Jew did significantly influence his personality. Anti-Semitism has existed for thousands of years in almost every corner of the world, but in Europe in the late 30's, it was reaching a height the world had never seen or I dare say has seen since, resulting in the Holocaust. As a teenager, Reggie experienced the bombing of London. Being aware of Hitler's attitude toward the Jews had to have some effect upon him as a young man. It appears that such was the case since he joined the military as soon as he was old enough. Reggie was not satisfied to be just part of the military establishment of Great Britain, he wanted to be the best he could be and ultimately earned a commission in an elite Highland Regiment which had rarely ever had a Jewish officer in its ranks. This desire to be a member of a respected group without changing who he was to do so (his race) is perhaps the first real glimpse we have into the personality of the man. We also have a glimpse of his leadership abilities. As a grade-school dropout he was not automatically sent to officers' training school but within three weeks his abilities were noticed and he began his officer's training. This task of fighting his way up from a position of disadvantage developed in his words, "a certain defensive determination to outdo everyone at their own game." The combination of defensiveness and determination that developed in the military are two qualities that have been important to his chiropractic career. Reggie has been placed or has placed himself in the position of defending chiropractic against antagonistic radio interviewers, against medical doctors in sometimes rather heated debates and unfortunately even against members of his own profession who object to the straight approach to chiropractic. While defensive, his words and actions are anything but meek and unassuming. He has always demonstrated an aggressive defense of chiropractic, determined that his point should be made very clear and most importantly, determined that his approach to chiropractic should survive. An aggressive defense combined with determination, whether in war or in a chiropractic debate, is difficult to overcome. These qualities developed in the military have been demonstrated throughout Reggie's career.

His race, coupled with his military career, also fostered the desire to be the best at everything he did and to strive for perfection in every area. The first in any organization, whether it be the first black baseball player like Jackie Robinson or the first Jewish officer in a regiment, is scrutinized under a microscope, and without a desire to be the absolute best he or she can be, will rarely succeed. This trait, developed in the army, has carried into Reggie's chiropractic career. He continually strives to perfect the philosophy, to make it more clear, more simple, more logical, more acceptable and more practical to all of society. He often says, "People are like cooked spaghetti, they can be pulled but they cannot be pushed." To pull you have to be out front, to be a leader. A leader is always striving to be better than everyone else and in so doing he makes everyone else better. Reggie's striving for perfection and desire to be the best at everything exemplifies that principle. Through that character quality he has made thousands of chiropractors better than they had ever hoped they could be.

I once asked Reggie why he was so strong in his position, why he took such radical positions in matters relative to chiropractic. He explained that people only accept 85% of what he says, so that if he watered down his message by even 10%, people would inevitably accept that much less of the message.

He describes himself as a "loner" in the military, an "outcast" because of his race. This must have been especially tough on him because elite military organizations are usually close-knit groups. He was feeling like an outcast because of his being a Jew in an organization which was fighting a country committed to destroying his race. While this ostracism was not apparent, it had a strong impact upon his personality and life. He has been able to do and say the things that he has said and continues to say because of his willingness to accept the loner and outcast role. But those two traits are important to a true leader. Perhaps these qualities, more than the ability and opportunity to command men, are what developed the leadership skill in Reggie. "It is lonely at the top" is more than a trite saying. Often leaders are outcasts, especially when they appear to have served their usefulness. Reggie's fellow countryman, Winston Churchill is a prime example. It has been said that leaders are born in a crisis. It may not be so much that a crisis brings out their leadership qualities, but that the qualities they have had all along are only seen as important in crisis situations. Once the crisis has passed, the leader, like Churchill, is no longer appreciated for those qualities. Reggie's ability to be a leader in the profession for almost thirty years must, in part, be his willingness to stand alone with his ideas and to be set apart because of them. (The need for leadership is also, in no small part, because the chiropractic profession has been in a continual state of crisis for the past thirty years and desperate for leaders!)

Part of the enigma of the man is manifested by the outworking of these qualities. True leaders do not really care what other people think about them, that is how they are able to stretch people's thinking and lead them. A military leader does not long for the friendship or love of the men he leads. A drill instructor does not take a Dale Carnegie course on "How to Win Friends and Influence People." His concern is that they respect his authority and follow his orders. But Reggie strongly desired the acceptance of his fellow regimental officers. Once, at a party, a group of officers were making some snide racial remarks. Reg invited the biggest and toughest to step outside. He won the respect of the regiment with that action, despite losing the fight that night!

Constantly striving for improvement has led Reggie to the underdog position and to the aid the underdog because life is not always fair. Whether taking on the toughest soldier in the outfit or in his role as the spokesman for straight chiropractic, to Reg there is no such thing as a lost cause. He has often said there is no such thing as an incurable disease until the patient is dead. Similarly, there is no such thing as a lost cause until there is no one left to fight for it. Reggie has never had a fear of being that person. His famous "obituary" speech given at a 1963 Palmer Homecoming, offers a glimpse of the man's willingness to be out in front all alone, taking on the most powerful enemies, including the two that hurt straight chiropractic the most, apathy and status quo. That obituary follows:

> **Headline: Last Practicing Chiropractor Dies at age 97** Today in Spring Valley, New York, Dr. Reginald R. Gold, Chiropractor passed away at age 97. He is survived by a wife who is also a chiropractor and retired from active practice several years ago. This ends an era in American history. Chiropractic started in Davenport, Iowa in 1895 and there followed a long and bitter struggle for survival against the combined might of organized medicine and the pharmaceutical industry. In the beginning it seemed as if the dedication and devotion of the chiropractors and the logic of their cause would be enough to overcome their monumental foe and to replace it as the world's number one healing art. But sometime during the 1960's or 1970's the tide gradually turned against the chiropractors. More and more chiropractors realized the hopelessness of their self-appointed task of saving the world. One by one they crumbled under the pressures of society and gave up fighting for their lost principle. They took instead the easier path of working for their personal acceptance and for status in the community. One by one their radical leaders died off or were deserted by their followers. And with each successive move away from their radical and unaccepted theories, the chiropractors became more and more a part of the established health team. Seven years ago in the year 2015 just 120 years after its birth, chiropractic officially died,

> as almost all of its remaining few practitioners were formed into a paramedical group to aid doctors of physical medicine in manipulation. A few who failed to qualify continued to practice illegally under their defunct chiropractic licenses. The last of these, Dr. Reginald R. Gold passed away last Monday. The funeral was unattended.

While Reggie on one hand appears to relish underdog causes and is not fearful of controversy, he very much desires to impress his fellow chiropractors and to earn their respect. That respect, however, must be on his terms. He will work to earn it but he will not compromise his principles to get it. He cares what others in chiropractic think of him as a chiropractor and strives for perfection to earn their admiration. When practicing, he wanted a larger practice than anyone. When teaching, he wanted to be the best and when lecturing, the most articulate. He works hard at everything he does but he does it so well that it looks easy. This is part of the complexity of the man. Reggie has a great need for acceptance. That may very well be some of the motivation to make his brand of chiropractic as acceptable as possible. Most straight chiropractors seem to have difficulty separating the philosophy from themselves because the chiropractic philosophy and practice is not just a job but a way of life. Consequently, when someone rejects the philosophy, a straight chiropractor often takes it personally. Apparently, Reggie feels this way as well. Reggie continually strives to convince everyone, chiropractors and lay persons alike, of the importance of straight chiropractic care. The straight chiropractic profession has directly and enormously benefited from it. Reggie has been motivated to distill the chiropractic philosophy into the simplest, most easily understood and accepted concept in the history of the profession. It is very fortunate that Reg has assumed that undertaking because at this point in history, chiropractic is coming under tremendous pressure and challenge from outside and within the profession, and its philosophy needs to be as clear and irrefutable as possible. Reggie has done just that for chiropractic.

Reggie has made some changes in his life over the years. At this time in his life he no longer sees himself as a rebel. At one time he was very anti-medical in his speaking and for a period of time he was also very anti-mixing. It may be that his experience with spinology made a significant change in him. As a spinologist, he was forced to take a totally neutral position relative to the health fields (remember Spinology is not a health field). As a result, he became very much less antagonistic toward medicine. This is quite a change for the man who helped promote bumper stickers in the early seventies that said, "My chiropractor says drugs are dumb, whether pushed or prescribed." He began to espouse the idea that "It's not our place to judge the value of, merit of or need for medicine." He also began to take a more conciliatory attitude toward mixing chiropractic, where he had previously been very anti-mixing. He once placed an ad in a sixties chiropractic school yearbook that said, "Chiropractic first, medicine second, surgery last, mixing never!" His position now became one of, "it is a legitimate way to practice chiropractic. It is just not the best way nor is it the way I choose." Unfortunately, many still perceive him as a rebel. He says, "A rebel is against things, I'm not against anything. I sometimes wish I could drag the rest of the chiropractors into seeing what chiropractic is, but that is not against anything."

I am not sure that he was ever a rebel. He loved the military life, which is about the most conforming life one could lead. He played soldier as a child and joined a cadet corp as a youngster, rising to its highest officer status. He was very happy with the structure of army life. While most people saw much of military life as a waste of time, Reggie had enough foresight to see the value of the structure, the discipline, the rote drilling, all to build an automatic response to command and to develop an efficient fighting machine.

While happy as part of the system, he was never reluctant to use the system to champion causes he believed correct. As a teenager he joined an organization called the 43 Group. It was started by Jewish servicemen who had fought Hitler in Europe and were now

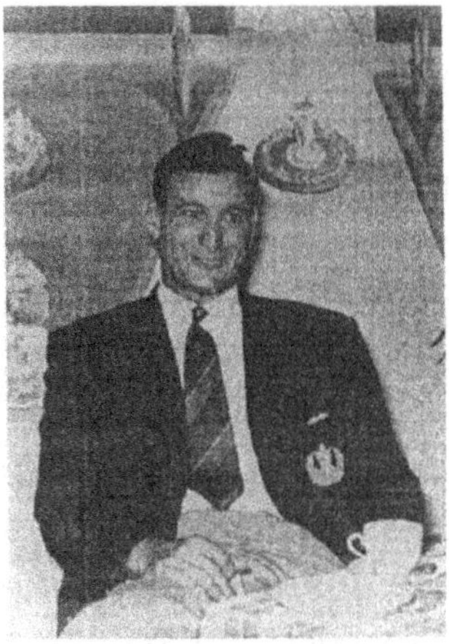

Reggie relaxing in a blazer that carried the emblem of his Highland Regiment

trying to make people aware of the fascist organizations in England. He was active with this group through his entire military career and often stood on one of the famous soapboxes in Hyde Park delivering a speech about the dangers of fascism. By doing so, he probably made one of Scotland Yard's "lists." These occasions may have been the first real demonstration of his speaking skills. Toward the end of the war, he was in the Desert Campaign where the famous German General Rommell, the Desert Fox, had gained his notoriety.

Later, Reggie was working as a liaison between the British Army and the Egyptian police trying to stop the drug trafficking that was occurring between some Egyptian civilians and British military personnel.

In this position, Reggie was able to help smuggle guns to the Jews in Palestine who were preparing to become the nation of Israel and knew that they would have to protect that sovereign nation status against the Arab world. At one point, Reg and his groups' activities were discovered by the Egyptian authorities. All escaped but Reggie who was taken to a Port Said jail where he was beaten by the Egyptians and suffered the first of several broken noses. Fortunately, he had become friendly with an Egyptian police official through his military role who was able to get him freed. Actually, the Egyptian official came to the Port Said jail where Reggie was being held and bribed the jailers to release him.

On another occasion Reggie was given the command post of an immigrant internment camp in Cyprus for Jews emigrating to Israel. Just before his transfer, someone realized he was Jewish and his orders were immediately changed before he could use his position to help his fellow Jews.

Reggie left the military in 1948 and a year later he and his entire family left England for North America. His brother had been in the Royal Air Force and for a time was stationed in Canada. He convinced the family of the opportunities in the United States and so in 1949 Reggie found himself in America. His first job was as a pin setter in a bowling alley in Manhattan before the advent of automatic pin setting devices. Having no education and only military skills, there were few jobs for an English immigrant in New York at that time. Very quickly he decided that dodging errant bowling balls was not a good, long-term career choice and decided to put his communication skills to work by getting into sales. Reg sold door-to-door everything from encyclopedias to cemetery plots. Within a short time an old army friend came to the states and the two decided to go into a partnership in the antique business. They sold only to businesses and what they could not sell was sent to an auction house. Reg traveled to Europe where he would buy antiques and then ship them back to New York and return to New York himself. While he was selling the shipment, his partner was in Europe buying more. When he returned, Reggie would travel again. This experience gave Reggie a love for other countries, diverse cultures and a desire to travel. This has been helpful to him inasmuch as he travels almost 200,000 miles a year doing seminars in Japan, Australia, New Zealand and Europe, as well as across both the United States and Canada.

In addition to a love for travel, his former occupation gave him a love and appreciation for fine art and antiques that still continues today.

Reg's antique business was very successful. It was a business that most people would have made a happy, lifelong career. The opportunity to travel half the year, to see the cultural centers of the world and to make an extremely good living would be a dream come true for many. While Reg was very happy in his life, he admits that in the back of his mind he always thought that he would make a greater contribution to the world. Perhaps some of the important things he had already done in his life, making a contribution to the war effort and the fledgling nation of Israel, made him feel that there were better things in store for his life beside selling antiques. As he says today, "if no one ever bought or sold another antique, the world would hardly be the worse off for it."

For a while Reg thought about the law profession. He was attracted to the thought of helping people in need who could not help themselves, but it was at this time that he first was exposed to chiropractic. After coming to America, Reg developed severe allergies. By late fall, each year he had asthma-like attacks and was unable to sleep lying down despite taking numerous types of medication to relieve the allergy symptoms. A business acquaintance suggested he try a chiropractor. Reg recalls that his first exposure to chiropractic was this fellow saying, "You may think I'm crazy for saying this, but have you considered a chiropractor?" His first introduction to chiropractic was associated with the idea of being crazy if you go. But if that was not enough, his actual experience with the chiropractor can only be described as somewhat bizarre. The address Reg was given in East Orange, New Jersey had no sign, just a street number and a doorbell. It was 1954 and chiropractic was illegal in New Jersey. He rang the doorbell and a pair of eyes peered out through a slot in the door like an old-time speakeasy. The voice behind the door said, "What do you want?" "I came to see Dr. Peruso," Reg replied. Dr. Frank Peruso, like other chiropractors in those days, was apprehensive about seeing new patients. It was common for the authorities to send a "plant" to a chiropractor and then arrest him for practicing medicine without a license. So Dr. Peruso was understandably apprehensive when this unannounced stranger showed up at his door. Reg finally convinced him that he was a legitimate patient. Dr. Peruso explained to Reggie what he was going to do for him. Many people have wondered what was said to have turned Reggie Gold on to chiropractic and what was the chiropractor like who imparted to Reggie enough chiropractic to interest him in the profession. As Reg recalls it, Dr. Peruso's explanation was not especially dynamic. It was a one-on-one, report-of-findings type talk where the New Jersey chiropractor gave the usual chiropractic explanation of that period, namely "we have found the cause of your problem." But in addition to relating his allergies to the spine. Dr. Peruso also explained the concept of innate intelligence and the idea of the balance of nature and how chiropractic related to those concepts. It was B.J. Palmer chiropractic. He related subluxation to the cause of DIS-EASE and DIS-EASE as the cause of disease. It is not the straight chiropractic of today but Reg remembers well that it was a clear explanation of 1954 straight chiropractic as Dr. Peruso knew it and practiced it. While Dr. Peruso related to his allergies, Reggie had enough of a vision to see how chiropractic could relate to all aspects of health problems. Dr. Peruso explained innate intelligence, the balance of nature and correcting cause.

Reg had a visionary idea of chiropractic even then. Most chiropractors were seeing very few patients for very few conditions. Reggie saw chiropractic applicable to every person with every condition. Of course that is not Reggie's vision of chiropractic today, but back then in the context of chiropractic getting sick people well, it was quite a bit for a first-time patient to grasp especially in twenty minutes or so. Reggie is truly one of those people who was turned on to chiropractic by its philosophy. Many people who ended up in chiropractic school in that period did so because chiropractic had drastically changed their health. Reg never even gave chiropractic a chance to improve his allergies. He received only one or two adjustments and three days later he was on his way to what was then the Palmer School of Chiropractic. Reg wonders whether he would have gotten into chiropractic had he seen "miraculous results." As it turned out his allergies did not improve for many years and anyone who has been to Davenport, Iowa in the summer knows that it is terrible for allergy sufferers. Often chiropractic results get in the way of an individual's philosophical understanding. Their thinking can go no further than the relief or seeming miracle cure they have experienced. That is why so many chiropractors cannot get out of the bad-back type practice. The results they get just continue to perpetuate those type of patients coming in the office and that type refers that type only, never sending in healthy people. Their entire focus is on the pain and its alleviation and that is all chiropractic ever is to them. Reggie's thinking was not clouded by results. He was free to think about the philosophy and its wide range application rather than whether it would relieve his sneezing and watery eyes. Perhaps that was a matter of the man's mindset or perhaps it was just the chiropractic profession's good fortune that he did not go into Dr. Peruso's office with a condition that responded immediately. But Reg got into chiropractic because of its philosophy. It was that first day that Reg brought up to Dr. Peruso the idea of him going to chiropractic school. When Reg began to question Dr. Peruso about the educational requirements, the New Jersey chiropractor at first thought he was questioning the professional qualifications of chiropractors. That could not have been further from the truth. Immediately upon grasping this idea for his life Reg also wanted it for his life's work. However, he almost did not go to chiropractic school. A number of obstacles had to be overcome.

Dr. Peruso, after realizing Reggie was interested in chiropractic as a career, was anxious to help. He first took him to Atlantic States Chiropractic Institute in New York City where he was an instructor. Like most chiropractic colleges in the Northeast in those days, it was a small, rather shabby building with second-hand equipment that had been donated by chiropractors. It had a part-time faculty. Reggie was totally unimpressed with the place and told Dr. Peruso on the way back to New Jersey that he was having second thoughts about chiropractic as a career. Dr. Peruso responded that Reg did not have to go to Atlantic States but that he could go to his alma mater in Davenport, Iowa. He explained the facilities and the type of education that Palmer offered. It was much more attractive to Reggie. The problem was he would have to totally give up his business, pull up his roots and travel to Davenport. But that was not the least of his obstacles. When he called out to Palmer, they informed him that the next class was beginning in three days and that it was the last class enrolling that would not require a college prerequisite. But Reggie wanted to be a chiropractor and apparently Palmer wanted him as a student just as badly. The school told him that if he could come out right away, they could get him into that class. There was one more obstacle. Reg still did not even have a high school diploma! But

Palmer said if he could pass a GED exam when he got out there, he could still be enrolled in that class. So January 1955, barely one week after first hearing the word chiropractic, sixth-grade drop-out Reg Gold was sitting in class at Palmer School of Chiropractic, preparing to become one of its most notable graduates.

Reg Gold had a "fun life," as he describes it, prior to chiropractic: traveling, living the life of a bachelor, making lots of money and not working hard at all. But his life had no purpose. He always believed that eventually his life would serve an important purpose. Besides the legal profession, he had thought of being an investigative journalist. But when Dr. Peruso explained to him this different and unique approach to health, he knew what he would be doing the remainder of his life. It was a simple idea that he believed the world was ready for and he wanted to give up the good life he had to pursue a better life, not necessarily better in lifestyle or financially but better in purpose.

Preparation for the Profession

The Palmer campus in the mid 50's, by chiropractic standards back then, was impressive, far more so than the run-down buildings that were the schools in New York. The facilities were great, but the atmosphere was even better. B.J.'s active involvement was winding down but his presence still strongly permeated the school. The epigrams were still there covering almost every foot of wall space in the buildings. The animal heads were still there, as well as the vast osteological collection. There was the aura of the Palmers and the moment by moment realization that you were truly at the Fountainhead of Chiropractic. To Reggie this was what an Ivy League school should look like and he was thrilled to be a part of it. The students at Palmer were there for basically the same reasons as students in every generation: some because their health had been radically changed for the better under chiropractic care, some for humanitarian reasons, some because of an anti-medicine belief and some because they saw it as a way to make a very good living. Perhaps the only thing that has changed over the years is the percentage in each group. Today fewer students want to become chiropractors because they had a life saving experience, while many more see it as a way of making good money. There are two other types of students that Reg has seen over the past thirty years. The first includes the students who came to Sherman in the early seventies with a desire to change the world. They had gone through the turbulent sixties and experienced or had seen first-hand the frustration of that generation. Straight chiropractic represented a radical departure from the establishment (there is nothing more establishment than medicine) and also a practical way of changing people's lives and ultimately the world. The other category which is a relatively recent phenomena is the student who gets into chiropractic to get into medicine. There have always been students who wanted to practice an alternative to medicine in the treatment of disease. Some chiropractic schools were begun for precisely that purpose. But we now have students who want to be physicians and somehow see chiropractic as an avenue to reach that goal. Perhaps their desire has fostered the interest by one of the chiropractic colleges on the West Coast to add a medical curriculum to its program. That was definitely not Palmer College in the 50's. A number of students in that era, and their activities today, bespeak the typical student at PSC during Reggie's time there. They are some of the noted leaders in the profession. Five of the students attending PSC at that time eventually became presidents of chiropractic colleges: Reggie, Sid Williams, John Miller, Jerry McAndrews and Thom Gelardi. Also attending at that time was Chuck Gibson, a well-known practice management consultant. Joe Flesia, one of the founders of Renaissance, was also in the same class as Reggie.

Although Reggie had made good money in his antique business, living the good life did not include saving enough money to pay for his education without ongoing income. He had expected to stay in the antique business at least for a while so he had not financially prepared for Palmer or any schooling. Before he rang that bell of Dr. Peruso's office, he had not expected to be giving up his work and his income, moving to Iowa and assuming the lifestyle of a student. There were, of course, no student loans in those days, so Reggie, like thousands of other Palmer students during those years, had to work his way through chiropractic school. He started out living at the YMCA until he could afford an apartment. He took a job as a salesman but the time involved in that type of work and the conflict with his studies made it difficult. His social life consisted of playing cards on the weekends, eating popcorn and drinking Kool-aid at someone's apartment or house. On one of these occasions, he met a young lady and began dating her. She had a brother who worked part-time as a janitor at the Davenport Museum and he told Reggie he thought he could get him a part-time job there. Subsequently, he became the lowest paid assistant museum curator in the world making seventy-five cents an hour. Reggie's boss, the museum curator, worked with the Quad Cities Music Guild which put on musicals in the summer. That particular summer they were doing Bridgadoon and he asked Reggie if he would help out as a technical advisor with the actors learning their Scottish accents. There were not too many British accents in mid-western United States at that time. There was one speaking part in the musical that no one could seem to handle so Reggie was asked to play the part. Through that experience, one of the directors of the Guild who had a television program on Saturdays asked Reggie to work at the television station. He also found a Saturday night job as a radio disc jockey, playing a new kind of music that was starting to catch on called "rock 'n roll." Between those three part-time jobs and his studies, Reggie was kept very busy during his years at Palmer.

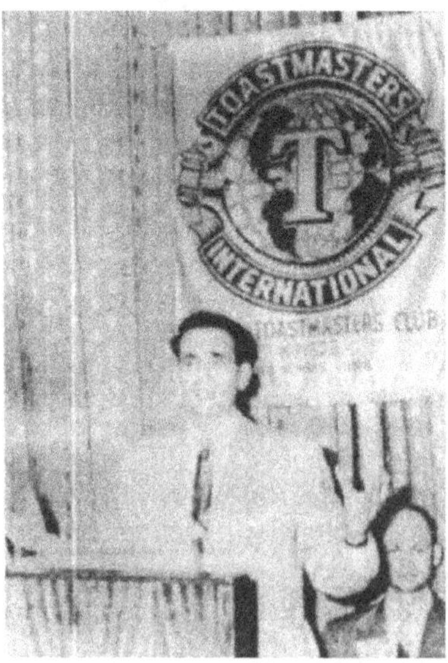

Winner of the 1957 Regional Toastmasters Speech Contest

Despite the heavy academic and work schedule, Reggie still found time to be involved in professional chiropractic activities that enabled him to use and develop his leadership and speaking skills. He was elected class president, no small feat considering the many outstanding personalities among his classmates. He was also the student representative to the International Chiropractors Association (ICA), whose president at that time was B.J.

But without doubt, Reggie's greatest passion, as he describes it, was what would be his hallmark in chiropractic, public speaking. He joined the local Toastmasters Club, an organization found throughout the world that teaches and gives opportunities for people to learn, develop and practice their public speaking skills. Reggie became president of the Toastmasters Club, won the local and regional competitions in speaking and was scheduled to go to the national championship in Dallas, Texas to compete against the winners from the other three regions of the country. However, final exams for his Junior year at Palmer prevented him from participating and the runner-up in the region went in his place.

The seeds of leadership that were planted in the military were nurtured at Palmer. However, Reggie never saw himself as a leader or set goals to reach positions of leadership in the profession. His goal was to excel, period. He wanted to be the best that he could be and to be better than his peers, in part to gain their acceptance. In this striving for excellence, to be the best, he naturally gravitated toward positions of leadership. First, because there are very few people in this world who strive for excellence. Mediocrity is the norm for most people. Individuals who excel realize that objective alone qualifies them for positions of leadership, even more so than others with better credentials, more experience or even greater ability. Not only does that quality motivate a person to leadership positions, but it also causes others to put them into positions of leadership. People want someone who will work hard to make an organization or a group the best it can be and someone who has that mindset for themselves will have it for the organization. Also, by electing that type of person, the membership can sit back and relax and, inasmuch as most people are lazy, it benefits them to have high achievers in position of leadership. Even at Palmer, Reggie was already one of those high achievers.

Not only did Reg not see himself as a leader in the chiropractic profession, he did not even see himself practicing chiropractic in the United States. Early in his career at Palmer, his plans were to return to England and practice on Harley Street in London. At the time, Harley Street was where all the top specialists in the country had their offices. Reg wanted to be among them, practicing straight chiropractic and demonstrating to the world that chiropractic was just as esteemed a healing art as anything medicine had to offer. He wanted, for himself and chiropractic, respect from the public and the other doctors. Practicing among them on Harley Street was a way to get that respect even though it might come reluctantly. As already mentioned, Reggie has always and continues to desire respect and admiration from friends, colleagues and even those that oppose him. Their friendship was not important, at least not as important as their respect, so whatever it took to gain respect he would do it. In school, that took the form of excelling in the academic arena.

His interest in academics is part of the complexity and enigma of the man. Reggie would be the first to agree that much of the education of a chiropractor is worthless to the practice of chiropractic and may even be detrimental to some people, in that it takes them away from the chiropractic objective. While the training in the mid-fifties was much more "chiropractic" than at CCE schools today, still much of it was of no value. Yet, Reggie excelled in his studies, not just philosophy but all his subjects. His feeling was that it was a course that had to be taken, and worthless or not, if you had to pass it, you should strive for not even just an "A" but an "A+." One instructor told Reg that because

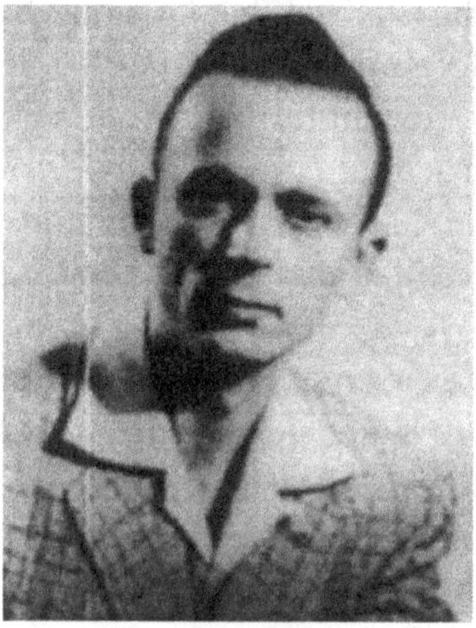

Rolf Peters
A roommate of Reggie's at Palmer

of his pop quiz grades he could skip the final and still get an "A" in the course. Reg opted to study for and take the final so he could get an "A+" in the myology course. He succeeded.

Reggie had a roommate through part of his time at Palmer, a German fellow named Rolf Peters. The two studied religiously and pushed each other to excel academically. Rolf, an outstanding student himself, is today a successful chiropractor in Australia.

While Reg was driven to excel in all his academic subjects, it was the philosophy that totally fascinated him. Of his four philosophy courses, he most fondly remembers those taught by Dr. Marshall Himes and Dr. Galen Price. When it came to teaching the chiropractic philosophy, Dr. Price was easily the most influential person in Reggie's student life. Reggie would sit in class totally enraptured by Price's presentation of the chiropractic philosophy. As it was unfolded to him in lectures, he was excited about, not the simplicity and beauty, but the complexity of the chiropractic philosophy, how it enabled people to excel, to be the best that they could possibly be, Reg's own personal goal. He could not understand how students could be totally ambivalent to or disinterested in the philosophy. He thought it was the most interesting and exciting thing he had ever heard and could not see how his classmates did not view it the same way. Dr. Price had the unique ability to apply the philosophy to everyday life. One particular example is still vivid in Reg's mind after almost forty years. Dr. Price was talking about innate intelligence and innate living. He explained that in raising his children he had an open refrigerator policy. The children could go into the refrigerator anytime they wanted, anytime they felt a desire for some food and eat whatever they wanted. He explained that his children were healthy and had developed good eating habits, innately, by their own efforts rather than educated by the efforts of the parents. This aspect of the philosophy impressed Reg. This was not just a health care philosophy but a way to live your life and to raise your children and to teach them or let them teach themselves a healthy lifestyle. The philosophy had tremendous ramifications and through Dr. Price's presentation of it, more than anyone else, Reggie Gold was turned on to a lifetime of living it, exploring it and sharing it with others. It is ironic that the complexity of the philosophy and the far reaching applications of it were what so impressed Reggie. Yet, his greatest contribution to the profession is his efforts in making that philosophy as simple as he can.

B.J. Palmer, while his force upon the profession was waning, was still an important figure on the Palmer campus. He was living in Sarasota, Florida, making only a few visits to Davenport each year. But B.J. was still B.J. and commanded the admiration and respect afforded the Developer and son of the Discoverer of Chiropractic. Students on campus who did not know him were either sent to Palmer by a parent or chiropractor who did and the aura of the man was passed along to this generation of students who were not privileged to hear him speak on a regular basis. He would address the student body a few times a year when business or a Lyceum brought him to Davenport. On one such occasion, Reggie, because of his speaking abilities, was given the privilege of introducing B.J. to the student body. In his introductory remarks, he talked of Palmer as being the future graduates' alma mater, the mother who nourished them in their understanding of chiropractic. He went on to say that if Palmer the school was their mother, then surely B.J. was their chiropractic father. From that time on, whenever B.J. would address Reggie, he would call him "son." Reg says it may be that B.J. couldn't remember his name. Even if that were the case I'm sure that B.J. would have been proud to have a son like Reggie. Contrary to the charges of many of Reggie's critics, however, Reggie is anything but a clone of B.J. Reggie has taken many of the concepts that B.J. introduced and developed and expanded upon them, just as B.J. expanded upon the original concepts of his father. One example is B.J.'s Utopia as presented in Stephenson's *Chiropractic Textbook:*

> "In accordance with the hopeful idea given by the Universal Cycle, Dr. Palmer's love for the human race and solicitude for the suffering, led him to hold that chiropractors have a great mission to perform.

> 'Not to improve the basic law - this is impossible - but to remove any negative obstructions brought about by perversions of that law, to the further end of a greater and freer expression of what the law of cycles demands in every phase and attribute.' If Chiropractic would be allowed to do this, an ideal state of affairs could be brought nearer. This state of affairs, which is not impossible for chiropractors to bring about, if they had the chance, would approach the ideal. An ideal state of sociology is a utopia.
>
> "An ideal sociological state would be a country or a world without sickness, insanity, blindness, feeble-minded people, deaf and dumb, backward children, social evils, criminality, drunkenness and its attendant evils, abnormal reproduction, and reasonable time allowed for the results to be brought about, it *could do much;* more than any other human agency has done or can do, in reducing the above named abnormalities to a minimum. This would be a great economic saving, because there could be fewer public and charitable institutions and penal institutions."

B.J.'s concept addressed sick people, physically or mentally. But Reggie took the basic idea and expanded it to include not only apparently healthy individuals but also the idea of improving ones potential in all areas of life. In my opinion, this may very well be the most important concept in chiropractic since its discovery. Without the application of this idea, chiropractic will undoubtedly degenerate into just a minor drugless treatment for certain conditions and definitely never reach the masses. The idea of chiropractic for everyone regardless of their health status, to enable them to reach their fullest potential in every aspect of life is a concept that can take chiropractic to universal acceptance. Despite the fact B.J. presented his "Utopia" concept in the 20's, it was not until the 80's that chiropractors began to make practical application of the idea and that was largely due to the efforts of Reggie.

Another concept that was touched upon by B.J., but never really applied until Reggie addressed it in the late sixties, was the idea of staying healthy with regular chiropractic care. The saying, "If you use chiropractic to get you well, you should also use it to keep you well," was known in those days but rarely used and rarely applied. Maintenance care was a logical outgrowth of chiropractic adjustments but for some reason it was never an important idea communicated by chiropractors. It demonstrates one of Reggie's major attributes. He has the unique ability to illuminate a concept that should be obvious to everyone, that is so simple and logical. Part of this is the ability to articulate truth in a simple and understandable way. Perhaps one of the most common observations from people who attend a talk given by Reggie is that what he has to say is so simple and logical that they can not understand why they did not realize it sooner. This observation comes from lay people, chiropractors and chiropractic students alike. The many testimonials in the introduction attest to the light that was turned on in peoples' minds by Reggie's speaking. These two concepts (chiropractic improves potential in all areas of life and staying healthy with regular care), developed and articulated by Reggie, are undoubtedly the two most important in chiropractic in the last fifty years, perhaps since D.D.'s initial discovery.

While Reggie has been unfairly accused of being a B.J. clone by many in the mixing aspect of the profession, he has also been charged with changing the philosophy as espoused by B.J. by some in the traditional straight chiropractic camp. These are the people who would like to camp at the grave side of our ancestors, who would desire to practice the same "chiropractic gets sick people well" model that B.J. purported a half a century ago. While it is a fair charge that he has changed that model, it is also true that the change was desperately needed to keep up with 21st Century health care and most important, to assure chiropractic a place in the future. He has made a few strong breaks with the chiropractic of B.J., however none of the changes Reggie has made or expressed are in any way contradictory to the philosophy that B.J. taught. The two most obvious changes are not philosophical at all. They address technique and chiropractic's relationship, or lack of relationship to medicine. Reggie abandoned the HIO concept developed by B.J. and became a full-spine practitioner. He also moved away from the anti-medicine rhetoric that was prevalent in B.J.'s day (and still is among many traditional straight chiropractors). Reggie's early years had been marked by the same opposition to medicine and medical practice but as time went on he came to the realization that if you attack medicine then you may well be associated with the medical objective of relating to disease, its treatment, prevention or cause. In a sense this break with B.J. was philosophical in that the straight chiropractic perpetuated by Reggie focused on DIS-EASE and separated it from disease. Others at the time (and some still) related DIS-EASE to disease.

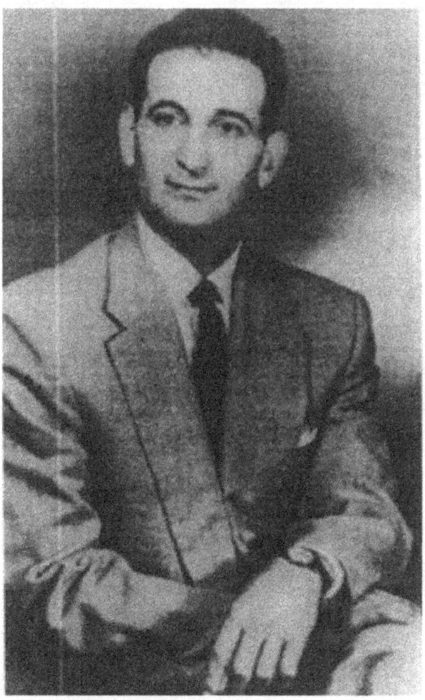

Reginald R. Gold, D.C.
Valedictorian and Class President,
Palmer School of Chiropractic

While Reggie had brief conversations with B.J. in the cafeteria, he acknowledges that his one on one conversations probably did not total more than one hour. Reggie's disagreements with B.J. did extend to conversations with him. One particular area where they had friendly disagreements was the confusion of universal intelligence and innate intelligence and the concept of "innate thot flashes." Reggie insisted that any "revelations" that did not come from the educated came from a cosmic consciousness connection, but by B.J.'s own definition of innate intelligence they were not innate. B.J. would actually kid Reggie about his insistence on keeping the terms separate and about their disagreement, but he never gave Reg the satisfaction of agreeing with him.

Reg has made some changes in B.J.'s explanation of the philosophy and has in many people's minds taken it to a greater and more acceptable level. In actuality, Reg regrets that it took him as long as it did to make these changes. It was only because of his reverence for B.J. and the philosophy that he developed as well as the school that he started that he didn't more readily change these concepts which were, in reality, hindering the growth of chiropractic. You cannot teach a philosophy based upon logic and deduction when there are certain aspects of it that are not logical. Reggie had to work with that handicap for a number of years. Finally he realized that the philosophy was bigger and more important than loyalty to a school or a man and that the man himself would want changes made if these were going to help further the profession. Changes were necessary if chiropractic was to reach any kind of universal acceptance. Holding to the traditional philosophy had only created a small group of B.J. loyalists while most of the profession moved further and further from the non-medical, non-therapeutic foundation of chiropractic. It was not until the late seventies that Reggie made what might be his most significant break from the traditional philosophy of B.J.'s, so it is obvious that for twenty-five years he was a strong proponent of it. Reggie started practice nearly believing that chiropractic could grow another arm on a one-armed man. "I totally believed who he (B.J.) was and I couldn't get past that until 1978." Standing on B.J.'s shoulders very much helped Reggie to gain the vision that he now has of chiropractic. But his avid respect and loyalty to the man and his philosophy also held him back from perhaps developing the philosophy much sooner than he did. Actually the ideas had been cultivating in his mind much earlier than the late seventies but out of respect to B.J. he was reluctant to share them with the profession. It was not until a significant event in 1979 that he felt free to expand his vision of chiropractic.

Reggie's days at Palmer were important. It gave him a deeper understanding of the philosophy, a way of looking at it deductively and ingrained in him the ADIO viewpoint of life. He further developed his communication skills and, of course, received a fine education preparing him for practice. In 1957, Reggie graduated from Palmer at the top of his class.

Reggie's Yearbook Message as Class President

> *The way has been long and hard, but we have learned well. Through the tireless efforts of our faculty we have learned to know and understand the chiropractic principle. We have learned consideration and tolerance for our fellow man. We have learned to overcome prejudice and to think objectively. We have learned humility in recognition of the existence of Innate Intelligence. Above all, we have learned how to learn.*
>
> *As we leave now to go our separate ways, we take with us this spirit of learning, a spirit which is the stronger because it is the product of no single mind, but rather the cumulative achievement of the energies of us all. Each of us donated a part of his cultural heritage to a common fund and each has received in return a share of that fund, so that, as we set out on our various pathways to success, our differences give us unity; our unity gives us courage; and our courage gives us strength to step proudly and confidently into the future.*
>
> *By God's will we entered to learn how. By God's will we go forth to serve.*

CHAPTER 2

Spring Valley Years

1958-1972

By his last year in chiropractic school, the idea of the London practice had been long forgotten. Reggie had come to the realization that getting chiropractic to the world was a better way to impress the medical community than by having a Harley Street, London office among them. While working as an intern at the B.J. Palmer Clinic, Reggie had met a wealthy Jewish businessman from Buenos Aires by the name of Jose Feldman who came to the Clinic for three months each year with his daughter who suffered with a neurological disease. Due to family and business obligations after three months the father and daughter would return to South America and return to Davenport nine months later. In talking to Feldman, Reggie convinced him that not only would it be better for the little girl to receive care twelve months of the year but also less expensive to have a chiropractor in Buenos Aires. Reggie proposed that if Feldman would set him up in practice and refer his wealthy friends and associates, he would learn the language and be that chiropractor. Feldman agreed to the idea. However, as Reggie's education was nearing its end, his letters to Feldman were being returned to him. From his limited ability to investigate the situation, it seemed that Feldman had disappeared. Whether his wealth had caused him to be a target of the government or some criminal element Reg could never ascertain. Only one thing was certain at the time, Reg was ready to graduate with no real plans for his practice.

While taking his final exams, Reg received a telegram that his father had passed away. His parents had been living in New York since arriving in the United States. His decision to take his finals rather than leave Palmer immediately for his father's funeral caused some friction in the family. After he finished his finals, he drove from Davenport to Livingston, New Jersey (a city in north Jersey not far from New York City) to see his mother who was living with his sister following his father's death. On the way to New Jersey, Reg's car broke down in the Rockland County town of Spring Valley, just north of New York City. He had only fourteen dollars in his pocket so he slept that night in his car. The next morning he shaved and bought a bus ticket to the next town - Pearl River. There he went to the office of Gerhardt Pepper, a chiropractor who Reg had met briefly as a student when he had introduced Dr. Pepper at a International Chiropractors Association function. Reg decided on the spot that Spring Valley would be as good a place as any to set up a practice. He told the elderly chiropractor of his plans and also that he had no money, and asked if Pepper could help him in any way. As Reg recalls it, "he reached into his pocket, pulled out a wad of singles and fives, peeled off $750 and stuck it in my hand."

Even with Pepper's generosity, opening a practice on $750 in 1957 was no easy task. Reg rented one half of a broken down drug store from an insurance man who had rented the building on the comer of Main and Church Streets and then realized it was more than he needed. He partitioned it for Reg, creating an L - shaped office. The longer leg of the L was 8 feet wide and 40 feet long. The shorter leg became living quarters with a shower and all the comforts an 8' x 15' home could afford. He bought a used card table from the Salvation Army for S2 to be used as his office desk and three folding chairs from the local funeral parlor for one dollar each. Reg had acquired a used spring-loaded Zenith Hi Lo Table, which did not work so he kept it locked in the down position as a stationary table. For $240 a month, Reg Gold had a home-office combination and officially began his chiropractic practice. By this time however, he had run up a debt of $5000. Most of the money was owed to plumbers, carpenters and electricians and for his x-ray unit. He went to each of the contractors and assured them that they would be paid every cent he owed them, but they would have to give him a little time. Further, he informed them that if they were really in a hurry to get their money they should start referring patients to his office.

He also decided to go to the local Jewish Center and join the young adult group to meet people, make contacts and build his practice. Unfortunately, they had no young singles group so he and another fellow organized one and planned a dance as its initial activity. The dance took place in September of 1958. A good number of people attended that dance including a young girl named Irene Siemens. Irene was working on her masters degree in nursing when she and a girlfriend decided to attend the dance. As Irene tells it, she and her girlfriend decided which guys at the dance they wanted to meet. Irene chose Reggie. She and Reg did meet that night and they began to date, and in April 1960, the founder of the young singles group no longer qualified for the organization. Irene was an RN when Reggie met her. She had worked both as a recovery room nurse and for the health department. Of course they had many long discussions about health, medicine and chiropractic. Despite her strong medical background, Irene understood and embraced chiropractic as Reggie explained it. She would accompany him in these early years, first as his girlfriend and then as his wife, to all kinds of chiropractic functions. Chiropractic was Irene and Reggie's social life. They would attend ICA functions and Irene became active in the Women's Auxiliary of the ICA. Of course that was at the time when Reggie and the ICA were alike in their thinking. Later, Reggie would move on in his philosophy and leave the ICA literally and philosophically. Irene would also accompany him to the philosophy

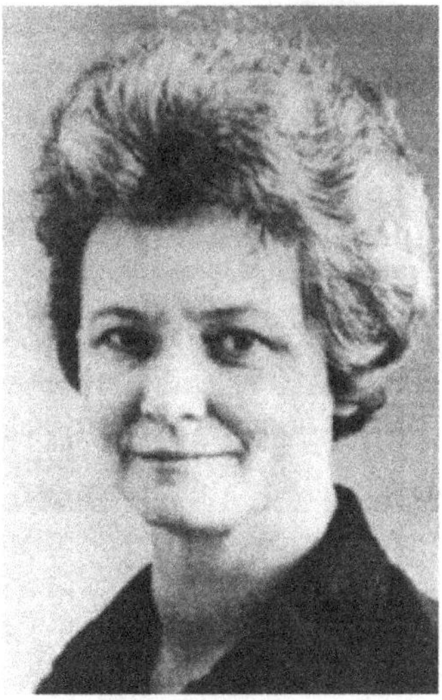

Irene Gold

sessions in upstate New York where the Bahans and people like Dan McGauern, Fred Lauro, Joe Holton of King, Ontario and Kenny Arsenault, a classmate of Reggie's, would get together and discuss the intricate and far-reaching aspects of the chiropractic philosophy. It was here and in discussions with Reg that Irene learned the chiropractic philosophy to the depth that she embraces it today.

Irene does not often get the opportunity to share chiropractic with large groups of people so not many people are aware of her understanding of the philosophy. Her present role in chiropractic gives her an opportunity to speak to many students from all the colleges in an informal atmosphere and to share chiropractic philosophy with them. Of course, having the last name of "Gold" elicits a number of questions from students who have only heard of Reggie and have never had the chance to hear him speak. She is able to stimulate interest in having Reggie to the school for a seminar (even if it need be "off-campus"). Irene helps promote Reggie's message by stimulating attendees at her board review courses with bits of straight chiropractic philosophy. But anyone who has had Irene as a teacher in chiropractic college knows the breadth of her understanding of chiropractic philosophy.

Irene admits that she has never been terribly comfortable up in front of a group of people. It was Reggie who encouraged her to be a speaker and a teacher. Although she has spoken to large groups of people, she is still much more comfortable in a teaching environment rather than on a platform. She had her first experience in communicating chiropractic to people in doing the new-patient orientations at Reg's office in Spring Valley, New York. Seeing hundreds of new patients each month necessitated that someone spend the hour or so that it takes to explain chiropractic to the new patient and, as was always the rule in Reggie's office, to his/her spouse. Reggie was away on speaking engagements much of the time and when he was at the office, he was busy adjusting people, so Irene assumed the task of doing the orientations and became, in her own way, an articulate and dynamic communicator. She, like Reg, was vitally involved in all aspects of chiropractic during their early years. On one occasion, while traveling back from a D.E. meeting where Reggie had just spoken, Irene said that although she had heard him speak hundreds of times, she realized that day that he was talking to her when he was speaking to the audience about becoming a chiropractor. The next semester she was enrolled in Columbia Institute of Chiropractic in New York City. It took thirteen years from their first meeting for Irene Gold to decide to become a chiropractor.

Irene Gold is a very special woman. She has been a faculty member at Sherman College of Straight Chiropractic and has served as Academic Dean. While teaching at Sherman, Irene began doing board review courses for the students. Before long, chiropractic students from all over the country were clamoring for her services and today Irene Gold Associates is the most successful board review course in the profession. There are thousands of chiropractors who owe their passing of state and national boards to Irene's tutelage. As a wife to Reggie, Irene has been an invaluable asset to his life's work. She has supported him 100% in every endeavor. Reg himself acknowledges that whether he was right or wrong she has always been totally loyal to him. That takes a remarkable person because many of the things Reggie has done over the years were ground breaking endeavors and occasionally put himself, his finances and his wife out on a limb. Leaving a successful practice to help begin the first new chiropractic college in almost twenty-five years is enough of a challenge for any one lifetime. But then to uproot yourself again and move from South Carolina to Pennsylvania to begin another school, then start Spinology, and constantly travel worldwide would be a strain on any spouse. But Irene has accepted it and has supported Reg through each of these endeavors even to the point of assisting him in the work associated with them. Much of Reggie's success has to be in good part due to the loyalty, support and help of Irene.

Promoting the Practice

When Reg began practice in 1958, the practice of chiropractic was still not licensed in the state of New York, so obviously he could not advertise in the traditional way (e.g., newspapers, yellow pages). However, just because he could not advertise does not mean he did not promote chiropractic. In fact, he promoted it heavily. His emphasis was upon how great chiropractic was and how bad medicine was. He was convinced from the traditional straight chiropractic philosophy that subluxation was the cause of all disease and that if medicine kept people from having their subluxations corrected (by keeping them out of chiropractic offices) then medicine must be bad. His strong position caused concern among some chiropractors who were trying to get chiropractic licensed and wanted the help of, or at least no interference from, the medical community. One of his good friends actually encouraged Reg to try to tone down his message. It is important to note, that when Reg now speaks against this idea of chiropractic getting sick people well or as an alternative to medicine, he speaks from the vantage point of having been there at one time himself.

Reggie admits that it took him a long time to stop the attack on medicine, even after he stopped presenting chiropractic as an alternative to medical care. He did it on the basis of knowing that there is no way the body could recover normalcy and balance if chemicals in the form of drugs are continually pumped into it. The other reason he continued the attack was a political one. If the people in the community believed that medicine was good then they would also believe the position that medicine held for almost three quarters of a century, that chiropractors were quacks. Attacking medicine still perpetuates the idea that chiropractic is an alternative. That is one of the most unfortunate images that chiropractic has projected over the years. Sadly, while Reggie and most of the objective straight chiropractic community have completely abandoned that idea, traditional straights (e.g., the ICA) have not.

Patient education was an important part of Reggie's practice from the first day. A new patient was always required to bring in his or her spouse for the new-patient orientation. Reg maintains that there is no way the entire family will be under chiropractic care unless both spouses fully understand the chiropractic objective. To expect a husband or wife to explain to his or her spouse in five minutes what it takes a chiropractor one hour to explain is unreasonable. They just cannot do it. So very early in his practice Reg began requiring that the spouse also attend the new patient orientation.

One of Reg's early endeavors was running a bus route through Spring Valley to bring patients into the office. He purchased a small school bus, had it painted gold, and ran it twice a day through the community. Like many suburban towns, Spring Valley had no public transportation. So he went around town and put up small signs designating bus stops. He recalls that he never bothered to ask permission. As he later related it, "Every bureaucrat is faced with a choice. They can either say no and make one person unhappy or say yes and run the risk of getting in trouble, so they always say no. The clerks always say no, so I just did it. If they had ordered me to take it down, I would have, but they never did." Dr. Jay Kaufman, a Cleveland graduate was Reg's primary bus driver until he was able to get into practice. Today, Jay is a successful straight chiropractor in Pennsylvania and a well-known chiropractic speaker in his own right. The bus offered many people an opportunity to get care who might not otherwise. There was a large Hasidic Jewish community in Spring Valley. Many of the men worked in the diamond district in New York and would go into the city every day leaving the family with no transportation. The Gold Bus provided transportation for them and many others in the area to get to the office and receive chiropractic care.

The bus did get Reg into a little trouble with the Chiropractic Board. Reg was never one to do anything part way and he enjoys being a little flamboyant. Prior to the bus incident, he had a run-in with the Board. Reg's stationery had a pair of embossed hands on it along with his name. They were no different than the hand emblems that you see everywhere except that along with his name and address the hands were gold. The Board claimed that he was inferring that he had "golden hands" thus holding himself out to be better than all the other chiropractors. They also saw the sign outside his office as misleading advertising. It read "Gold Chiropractic Office," rather than Reginald R. Gold. They were grasping at straws to find something on which to attack him. The bus, of course, was also painted gold and had Reg's name on it in large letters. The state board saw this as a clear violation of the advertising laws. The problem was that the state laws of New York required that a commercial vehicle have the name of the owner printed on the side of it. So state law said his name had to be on the bus but the Board declared it blatant illegal advertising. They were clearly out to get Reg's license. Reggie took the whole thing rather lightly except for one occasion when it became rather serious. Apparently a jealous chiropractor turned him in for the bus and the sign and the state board filed thirteen counts against him. By the time it was picked up by the local paper, the story was so distorted that they reported that Reg had already been convicted and had lost his license. One of the charges that the newspaper printed was that Reg had been practicing under the assumed name, "Gold Chiropractic Office." Unfortunately, Reg was on an extended speaking engagement in South Africa at this time so Irene had to take all the flak and talk to the reporters. By the time Reg came back, things were in a state of total confusion. Even his patients, thinking he might have "skipped town," were wondering who he was. Any one of those charges if true could have cost him his license. Nothing came of any of it and of course, the article exonerating him did not appear on the front page. Instead, it was buried somewhere on page fifteen. To this day Reg feels very bad that Irene was forced to deal with all the negatives during this incident all alone.

As the practice grew, Reg expanded his hours to seven days a week. With the office open on Sundays, families were able to stop on their way home from church to get adjusted. However, when Reggie began to do seminars and lectures around the country he sometimes had to leave the office from Friday through Sunday, so he began to hire associates. A number of fine chiropractors got their start working as an associate for Reggie.

Reg's educational program evolved from "chiropractic gets sick people well" when he first got out of school, to the idea of preventing disease. His practice during the sixties and seventies took on the real purpose that reflects his presentation of chiropractic today. He came to the realization that with the myriad of causes of disease like environment, genetics and dietary factors, it is impossible to claim that chiropractic can prevent disease. He began to teach people that chiropractic can remove one interference (vertebral subluxation) to health, well-being and potential. It was then just a matter of communicating that idea to people so they could grasp the importance of regular chiropractic care. Distinct phases of the evolution of Reg's education program are evident as his vision of chiropractic changed. The first phase was the one that he came out of school with, that is, chiropractic get sick people well regardless of the disease. The second phase was if chiropractic cannot cure you, getting rid of subluxations, will at least keep you from getting worse. The third phase was chiropractic care for the entire family to prevent children from getting what their parents had. The fourth phase was chiropractic care for everyone to stay as subluxation-free as possible because they, in and of themselves, are bad. That phase was never really presented to the public in a formal manner until 1979 when Reggie started Spinology. Reg had the vision for this phase before he started Spinology, but due to his tremendous loyalty to B.J. and chiropractic, he never really presented it. While this concept represents an evolution of chiropractic it is also unquestionably a departure. It is as unlike B.J.'s chiropractic as a fluorescent light fixture is different from Edison's first light bulb.

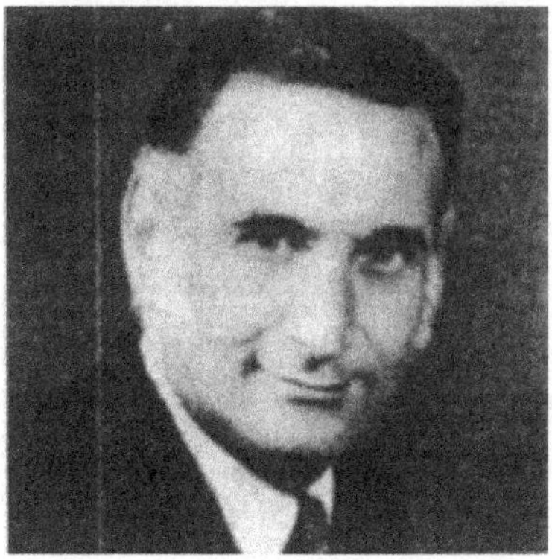

Columbia Institute

Reggie began teaching at Columbia Institute of Chiropractic in mid-town Manhattan in 1961. His reputation as a communicator was growing and he was willing to come into the city one day a week to teach philosophy. The fact that he refused to be paid for his teaching also made him a sought after faculty member. Columbia was started by a Dr. Frank Dean in 1919. While not necessarily a friend of B.J.'s, like Cleveland or Ratledge, Dean was supportive of straight chiropractic as it was practiced in the first half of the century. He was definitely opposed to the NCA (forerunner of the ACA) and its accrediting agency (forerunner of the CCE). The school was never large, occupying two brownstone houses in the middle of 71st street between Broadway and West End Avenue. The largest freshman class was 96 students in September 1964, the last year that students from New York could enroll without two years of college education. It was also the last year that Reggie taught. That, however, was an exceptionally large class. Most of the classes numbered between 12 to 15 students. Reggie felt that teaching was a way of giving back to chiropractic and he never accepted a salary for his time. This was always a matter of principle with Reg. He believed if you were in practice that alone should be your source of income and that teaching is an honor and a privilege and requires no remuneration. This idea worked great for Reggie. Of course, whether it is possible today with accrediting agencies and the extracurricular demands placed upon faculty is another question. While it might help to reduce the currently outrageous tuition costs, the colleges would probably not pass the savings on to the students. Reggie's idea of faculty working without pay did create some conflict for him later when he became an administrator at ADIO Institute of Straight Chiropractic. The basic idea is good. It creates a faculty, (at least the part-time portion of it) that is composed of successful chiropractors. These individuals are able to teach with more authority and to command more respect from students. Additionally, they have a wealth of practical experience to share with students, something that is sorely lacking at most chiropractic colleges. Many of the faculty at chiropractic colleges today cannot or chose not to be successful chiropractors. Often they are negative toward practice and are definitely not excited about it. These individuals hardly serve as good role models for students. At Columbia, there were many chiropractors who depended on the few dollars paid them for teaching to make a living but there were also a number of exceptions like Reggie, including Pasquale Cerasoli and later Jerry Witner and Larry Markson.

While this type of "gratis" faculty member may appear to be an asset to a college, he or she might not be appealing to the administration for various reasons. For example, it is true that a school would save money but they would also have to live with a person who did not "need" the job. Chiropractic tends to attract strong, independent people and many college presidents and administrators do not want that type of an individual working for them (usually because they are that type themselves). This was especially true in Reggie's case. As time went on, Reggie became both stronger in his convictions and more popular as an instructor. Consequently, he had occasion to run up against the then president of Columbia, Ernest G. Napolitano. "Nappy" was also strong in his convictions, although they seemed to change weekly. While he held to them, he held to them strongly. It was about this time that Columbia was moving more toward the ACA and mixing chiropractic and away from the ICA and straight chiropractic. This created clashes between Napolitano and Reggie, who had become very popular with the students. In fact, just prior to his taking a leave of absence, saving him the twice weekly trip to Manhattan from the suburbs, Reg held the position of Dean of Students. Reggie left because the school was not big enough for two strong personalities and Reggie would not back down from principle. While Napolitano could not keep Reggie on, he could not afford to lose the association of the increasingly well-known chiropractor from Rockland County. So his departure was called a leave of absence, although he never returned.

It was not only his teaching skills that created his popularity. In fact, his fame began to increase largely because of the tremendous practice that he began to build. After leaving Columbia, Reggie devoted himself to his practice. He scheduled a laymen lecture in April of 1965, the month he stopped teaching. In May, Irene recalls that the office signed up 256 new families as patients. That is not new patients but 256 entire families! People were starting to take notice of Reg, not just as an articulate philosopher but as someone who could build a volume practice. Irene says "We were working morning, noon and night, it was unbelievable." Reggie was doing all of the adjusting and Irene, while still not yet even considering a chiropractic career, was doing the new patient orientations. The following month Dr. Bert Dressier, another New York chiropractor began coming into the office three days a week to help out.

It was during his final days of teaching at Columbia that Reg began having what would become his very popular, Saturday night, philosophy sessions. The first ones were actually for the different classes at Columbia. Reg would invite the freshman class one month, then the sophomore class the next and so on. I have the distinct honor of being the first student to arrive for the very first of the Saturday night sessions. I misjudged the time it would take to get from Levittown, PA to Spring Valley, NY, and I and my girlfriend arrived two hours early. Those two hours before the others arrived and the evening talks turned the skeptical registered nurse with me into a lifetime proponent of chiropractic and my wife of over thirty years. After awhile, students started to come each month regardless of whose "mm" it was. From the beginning, spouses and girlfriends or boyfriends were always invited. However, some began inviting other friends and even field chiropractors. In those days, the mid-sixties, there were few seminars and there were even fewer people who taught philosophy, so the philosophy sessions became a monthly focus for many chiropractors. Lifelong friendships developed during the meetings. They usually began by 8 p.m. and sometimes did not end until the sun came up when the remaining attendees adjourned to a diner for breakfast.

There was no charge for the sessions; Reg gave of his time and energy to anyone who wanted to come. Bringing a box of donuts or a bag of bagels was appreciated but not required. It was not uncommon to have better than one hundred people crowded into Reggie's large family room that adjoined his chiropractic office. On one occasion over two hundred people were in attendance, some sitting upstairs in the dining room and living room straining to hear Reg downstairs. Furniture was pushed back against the walls and folding chairs were set up. Latecomers often had to sit on the carpeted steps going up to the dining room. Fortunately for the tropical fish, the large tanks were built right into the wall of the room. The waiting room would be stockpiled with cakes, cookies and bagels and cream cheese for the three or four breaks during the evening talk. There was good fellowship, food, plenty of coffee (you rarely saw Reggie without a mug of coffee in his hand) and an opportunity to share and get your spine checked in one of the adjusting rooms.

But the biggest attraction was Reg. He stood up in front of the group with his foot on a chair and just talked chiropractic philosophy for hours on end. He may not have been as articulate and dynamic as he is today, but he was the best by far that anyone in the Northeast had seen in years and that many had ever seen. There are many well known chiropractors who learned their philosophy at these sessions. Joe Flesia came down from Rhode Island to attend. Dick Plummer was not yet even in chiropractic school, but attended each month, brought there by his field chiropractor, Jim Doherty who had been a student of Reggie's at Columbia. Plummer describes his first exposure to Reggie in the Saturday night meetings.

> *"I was invited by Jim to go up to Reggie's on Saturday night. I had no idea who this guy was. Knowing that I was going to hear this famous doctor (my chiropractor's professor), I kept asking Jim, 'What am I going to wear?' He would reply 'Wear whatever you want.' Not knowing whether to wear a suit or not, I wore a sweater over a dress shirt and left a tie in the car in case everyone else was wearing ties. I got there and the place was packed. Down comes Reggie wearing bell-bottom denims; no socks; red, white and blue sneakers and a denim shirt that said, 'Property of Georgia State Prison.' Of course, he had the mutton-chop sideburns, long hair, although not as*

> *long as when he went to Sherman, and he was wearing massive amounts of turquoise jewelry and he had a giant coffee cup, it must have held a half gallon of coffee. They rang a little bell and got started. I sat there and listened to him go through the 'Triune of Life' and he was scribbling on the board drawing a line with 'doctors of therapy' on one side and 'doctors of cause' on the other, 'DT's and DC's.' I sat there as a patient listening to all of this. It started making sense and sinking in. So I started going back every month to listen to him. I would stay late talking to Reggie, Flesia, Irene or whoever stayed around to the early morning."*

Jim Sigafoose would travel to Spring Valley from a south central Pennsylvania town where he was developing a straight practice, having some years before graduated from National College. Another student who attended the monthly session was Dr. Joe Donofrio, who has been a high volume practitioner for almost thirty years, as well as chairman of the board of both Sherman College and the FSCO. Like many others, Joe benefited greatly from the monthly sessions, which lasted eight years until Reggie left for South Carolina. However, Joe's real introduction to chiropractic, like Doherty, myself and others, was in the classroom. In a letter to Reggie, informing him of Sherman College's desire to dedicate a building in his name, Donofrio expresses his feelings for what he learned from Reggie in philosophy class at Columbia.

> *"More than 30 years ago I left the campus of Seton Hall University for a small brownstone on the west side of New York City. During my first week of classes at Columbia Institute of Chiropractic, I was given pause by the lack of facilities and unprofessional attitude of my instructors. Perhaps I made a poor career choice. Perhaps chiropractors were frauds and quacks! Then, on Thursday afternoon, I attended a*

Chiropractic Philosophy course taught by Dr. Reg Gold. Dr. Gold began to weave a tapestry of exotic silks and pure gold for me with his words. A tapestry of chiropractic which he would continue to weave for the rest of my professional life, and I knew that I had not only found a career -I had found a life!"

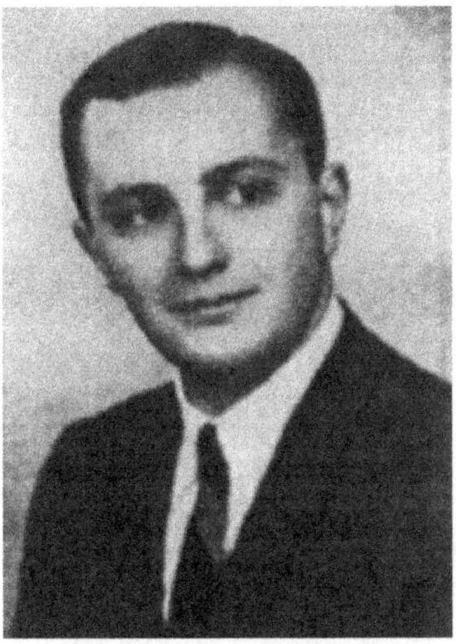

Joe Donofrio as he looked when a student of Reggie's at Columbia

There were many others who were touched by Reggie's speaking, both in his classroom lectures and the philosophy sessions in his home. Most are not well known, they are just good straight chiropractors who are taking care of thousands of people and who have themselves inspired countless others to go to chiropractic college.

Reggie's mission has always been to get the message of chiropractic out to people. To him, it mattered little whether it was a lay person, a chiropractic student or a practicing chiropractor. As an instructor at Columbia, the students were his primary focus. However, in the monthly meetings at his home, the field chiropractors became more and more the majority. In the mid-sixties, chiropractic was perhaps at its lowest point in its history. Estimates were that there were only about 14,000 chiropractors in the country. By 1967, the Chiropractic Institute of New York was closing and Lincoln College in Indiana was only a year or so away from closing. That would leave Columbia National College and Columbia as the only two chiropractic colleges east of the Mississippi.

There was very little enthusiasm in chiropractic and much less self esteem among chiropractors. So Reggie's message attracted many philosophy-starved practitioners to Spring Valley. He was always looking for other ways to communicate the spoken word about chiropractic. From his soapbox days as an 18-year-old in London, he realized he had a special gift in public speaking. He was talking to Kiwanas, Rotary Clubs, church groups or anyone who would invite him to speak. It was having an effect upon his practice, bringing in new patients, but he wanted more. At this time, he came in contact with a student, Russ Werner, whose father, the late Dr. Bill Werner, had been one of the most famous chiropractors in New York and a friend of B.J.'s. He had been a great motivator of lay people, having founded the American Bureau of Chiropractic and once filled Madison Square Garden with lay persons to hear B.J. and others speak. What struck Reggie was Dr. Werner's widow, Bernice's stories about the New York chiropractor's lectures to the public, bringing patients and interested people together and then explaining chiropractic to them. Dr. Werner had built one of the largest practices on the East Coast and lay lectures were in no small way a part of that success. With his love for public speaking and his obvious gift for doing lay lectures, this was a perfect vehicle for Reggie. No longer would he have to speak at a Rotary club or as an after dinner speaker between the dessert and the business meeting. From now on he would explain chiropractic to those people who had come to hear him lecture on the subject. Dr. Werner was Reggie's inspiration and motivation to do laymen lectures.

He privately lectured to his patients and those they brought to his talks. However, about this time, some of his students at Columbia were graduating and opening practices. They began to ask him to come to their office and lecture to their patients. He once traveled to Newburgh, New York, a trip that took three hours because of a blinding snowstorm, to speak to the patients of a former student, Jerry Witner. The only person to show up in the storm was Dr. Witner's mother so Reggie gave his full lay lecture for just her. For those chiropractors who have struggled with getting people to attend their lay lectures, it may be encouraging to know that even Reggie Gold had one where only one person showed up. Of course, the next month he went back and Jerry had packed his office with patients to hear

Reggie. Dr. Jerry Witner himself became an instructor at Columbia and is still a successful straight chiropractor in Newburgh.

Two other students of Reggie's, Pat and Walt Heaney, opened an office in Wappinger Falls, New York. For three straight months Reggie would go to their office and lecture to their patients. Finally on the third month, when he got up to speak, he said, "I would like to introduce a special guest speaker this evening, Dr. Walt Heaney!" Walt was initiated into doing lay lectures very quickly. From a practical standpoint, teaching and motivating chiropractors to do lay lectures may very well be Reggie's greatest contribution to building practices. Reg did not originate the lay lecture but he most assuredly refined it to its most simple, yet powerful format. What he was able to do for thousands of young practitioners was quite remarkable. Almost every chiropractor who heard him do a lay lecture would say the same thing, "I could never give a lecture like that!" On the one hand, they were awed by his ability and their own comparative inadequacy, while on the other there was something in his talk that made them say, "I want to try doing lectures myself." You may be overwhelmed by the confidence, the enthusiasm and the beauty of Reggie's delivery which The classic "foot on the chair" pose makes you feel like you could never give a lecture like that, but the simplicity of his message makes you realize that you should and could deliver the big idea to patients that chiropractic is so simple, so logical and so important that it does not matter how poor your speaking skills, you can communicate chiropractic to the average lay person and build a practice. Despite his extraordinary speaking skills, Reg was able to convince many young chiropractors that they

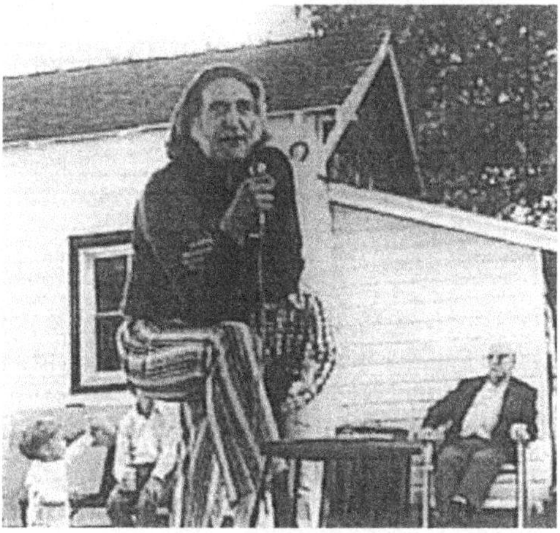

The classic "foot on the chair" pose

could easily do the same thing. Almost without exception, the most successful chiropractors of the last three decades are people who do lay lectures, whether they call them that or not, and I would venture to say that the vast majority of them use at least something from Reggie's lay lectures.

Of course, the fact that Reggie began to build an extraordinarily successful practice in Spring Valley was a major reason why young chiropractors wanted to do what he was doing. They felt if they could do a lay lecture only half as well as Reggie, they could build a practice half as large as his and still be successful beyond their wildest dreams. As his practice grew, his fame spread and his Saturday night philosophy sessions became packed houses! Early in Reggie's teaching career, Napolitano asked him to speak in his place at a state meeting. This was his first exposure to speaking to groups of chiropractors which would eventually be his most important contribution to the chiropractic profession. He began to speak at seminars and conventions and chiropractors wanted to hear the man who had built a practice of more than a thousand patients a week and was still growing!

Reggie's really big exposure to chiropractors, or more correctly their exposure to him, came through the D.E. (Dynamic Essentials) meetings started by Sid Williams in Atlanta, Georgia. Sid invited Reggie to come as a guest speaker and he quickly became the most popular speaker on the platform. During the course of the Thursday through Sunday seminar, Reggie would speak as much as five or six hours. Other speakers would lecture for one or two hours at most. The room was always packed. Even with five or six hours of Reggie on the platform, it was not unusual for 100 or 200 young chiropractors, their spouses, and C.A.s to sit around in a meeting room until one or two in the morning listening to Reg, long after the formal part of the program had ended. These were some of his most productive meetings, for it was here that he was able to field questions from the group in an informal atmosphere. As articulate and forceful as Reg is as a public speaker, he is perhaps at his best in an informal setting, doing a question and answer session. During these sessions, he would take question after question, for hours on end, never backing down, never dancing around the question and always bringing it back to chiropractic philosophy. It was in these meetings that many realized that Reggie was not just an articulate orator. He had a deep understanding of the chiropractic philosophy and was able to quickly draw from that knowledge to answer any and all questions. Chiropractic philosophy was quickly falling out of favor in the colleges in those pre-Sherman days and many chiropractors learned more chiropractic philosophy in an Atlanta hotel meeting room than they ever learned in chiropractic school. The audience for those midnight sessions often included a number of the other speakers on the platform. As well-known as they were, many of them could still learn from the man with the bushy side bums, standing in the middle of the room with one foot on the seat of a chair.

D.E. was good for Reggie. It gave him a tremendously larger audience than he had previously had. It exposed him and his philosophy to chiropractors from all over the United States rather than just the Northeast. Reggie was also good for D.E. He was a tremendous attraction. Many chiropractors came just to hear Reggie. With his late night talks, you might hear him for as many as eight to ten hours.

During Reggie's talks, he was not hesitant about being critical of non-chiropractic things and other speakers who gave a mixed message. He was also critical of the Si Nel Company, Sid's chiropractic supplier business, which sold stethoscopes and sphygmomanometers at the D.E. meetings. In 1971, a particular incident occurred that drastically affected Reggie's relationship with D.E. and Sid Williams. Reggie got up to speak after Dr. Nelson Peet, a fellow New York chiropractor had spoken. Peet was a Concept -Therapy practitioner, a philosophy begun by a Dr. Thurman Fleet in the 20's. Concept Therapy is based primarily on the power of positive thinking, only the particular practitioner was supposedly communicating these positive concepts to a patient's innate intelligence. Unfortunately, this is incompatible with chiropractic philosophy. We do not communicate anything to the innate intelligence of the body, nor does it need our puny, educated brain to help run the body. Well, when Reggie got up to speak, he began erasing the blackboard behind him and said something to the effect of "Let's get this concept-therapy garbage off the board." After the meeting, Sid and Reg had a disagreement over the appropriateness of Reg's remark. Sid did not want Reg to criticize other speakers, which is a reasonable position, but on the other hand, Reggie had to feel tremendous frustration, pouring so much energy into getting these chiropractors to understand what chiropractic was all about and then having that effort undermined by other speakers. It was clear that while D.E. was the best vehicle for Reg to get his message across, it simply was not lined up with his objective. More and more, D.E. was bringing in non-straight chiropractors and even non-chiropractors, including people in the field of nutrition and motivational speakers. As a result of the disagreement, Reggie was not invited to speak at the next D.E. meeting. He fully expected it to be a "one-meeting suspension" and kept his calendar free for future D.E. meetings. He was never invited back.

Reg's departure from D.E. affected both him and the D.E. program. He lost a major audience four times per year, but more importantly, the "D.E. movement" lost the philosophical, stablizing force that Reggie brought to the meetings. They lost many good, solid, straight chiropractors who no longer attended or supported Sid, D.E. or its goals. These were some of the most successful straight chiropractors in the profession. It is likely that the loss of Reggie and his "followers" was to some degree responsible for the D.E. movement's drift away from straight chiropractic, ultimately resulting in a major split between the traditional straight chiropractors which are today represented by Williams, D.E., the ICA and Life College and the objective straight chiropractors represented by Reggie, the FSCO and Sherman College.

As a result of his exposure at D.E., Reggie was becoming more in demand as a speaker at conventions and seminars. During this time, he still had the practice in Spring Valley. By the early seventies, it had become the largest practice in the United States, probably the world. The office was open seven days-a-week and besides himself, there were usually two other chiropractors on staff to cover the office while he was off speaking somewhere. Of course, Irene was doing orientations in addition to attending classes at Columbia Institute of Chiropractic. The practice was ever expanding, which is pretty remarkable considering the frequency with which Reggie was away. Anyone who has built a practice knows how difficult it is to do when the primary doctor is not present. The fact that the patients came despite Reggie's frequent absence, certainly speaks of the quality of the chiropractors he had working for him. But even more, it is an indication of his patients' understanding of chiropractic. They were not drawn just to the man, but to the message that said they needed to have their spines checked regularly regardless of who was on duty. They were faithful to chiropractic. This is the desire of every straight chiropractor. To know that the patients are not just attracted to your personality, but that they understand enough about chiropractic that should another chiropractor suddenly step in and take over the practice, they would still come regularly.

Reggie's fee system was as unique and as sensible as his message. When he opened his Spring Valley practice, he placed a "box on the wall." This was a modification of the old GPC (God-Patient-Chiropractor) system developed by Dr. George Shears and made famous by his nephews, the Bahans of Derry, New Hampshire. Reggie presented to his patients the idea that chiropractic was too important to put a price on it and that regular, lifetime care for the entire family necessitated a fee structure that was affordable to the patient. For this reason, each patient determined his or her own fee and placed it in a receptacle in the adjusting room. This was just one more way in which the patients realized the importance of regular adjustments. There were just three requirements to participate in the Cooperative Practice Program, as Reg called it. The patient had to come regularly, they had to attend a new patient lecture with a friend or spouse and of course, they had to refer others into the office. Reggie affected numerous chiropractors with this system and during one period there may have been as many as fifty chiropractors in the

New York, New Jersey and Pennsylvania area who had "box-on-the-wall" practices. Joe Donofrio and I are still practicing that way as a direct result of Reggie's influence. It is interesting that Reg has since changed his approach to fees. From his years of experience he felt that too many people did not utilize the fee system because of pride. Patients did not come if they could not afford to put at least something in the box. And no matter how much he explained that fees should not get in the way of an individual's health, the pride of many people kept them away. He now advocates a system in which the patient pays a yearly fee (to be determined by the chiropractor) at the beginning of care, and receives a discount for paying in advance. He believes that this system will allow the patient to be more regular and that they will not be reluctant to come in during a week when they are short on funds because they have already paid. Another advantage of this system is that it locks the patient into a longer initial care period and gives the chiropractor more time to educate them to lifetime care and for them to see the personal benefits of regular chiropractic care.

PACE

It was about the time that Reggie was at the height of his D.E. speaking that he began the Patients Association for Chiropractic Education (PACE). Again, Reggie took his lead from Dr. Bill Werner and his American Bureau of Chiropractic (ABC). The main objective of the ABC was to gain rights for chiropractic patients, the most obvious of which in Werner's day was the right to get adjusted. New York had no chiropractic licensing law so that was the focus of the ABC. While the organization never achieved the licensing objective and ceased to be a viable organization shortly after the death of Werner in 1959, the effect of exposing the public to chiropractic was an important side effect of the main objective. In fact, it may have been more important then the objective itself. This was especially true of PACE. Chiropractic licensing was won in 1963 in New York state, but there were still some restrictions on chiropractors such as not being allowed to x-ray below the level of the first lumbar. Probably the greatest restriction at this time was the inability of chiropractors

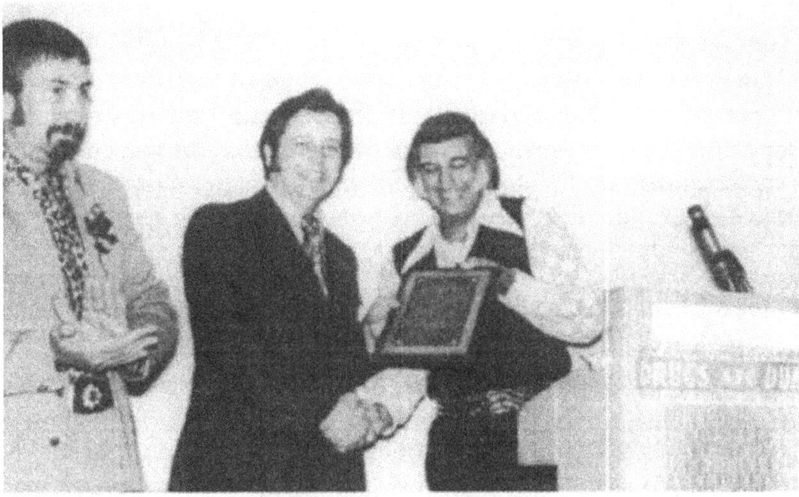

Reggie presenting an award to Kick Plummer at a Pennsylvania Chapter Fellowship Banquet in 1972, To the left is Jim Sigafoose

to advertise in New York State. This was the crusade of PACE.

It was ironic that in using a lay persons organization (as opposed to the individual professional) to fight the anti-advertising laws they accomplished both objectives. PACE not only educated the public to chiropractic, but they legally circumvented the state anti-advertising laws. Reg was involved in some very interesting situations as the State board questioned him about the ads that PACE was running. But PACE had its own officers, none of whom were chiropractors, Reggie was just the advisor and the chiropractic ads that were placed never advertised his office. They were paid for entirely by PACE which organized a variety of events to raise funds. All of their ads included an invitation for anyone and everyone to attend their monthly meetings The fact that the meetings were held at Reggie's home-office and the fact that Reggie gave a lay lecture at each meeting was just coincidental. Everything was legal and legitimate which frustrated both the State board and the mixers in the area.

The state board was barely able to restrain the chiropractors' freedom of speech. They knew they had no chance of muzzling lay people in light of the First Amendment right to freedom of speech. The idea was brilliant. The message was getting out and it was being paid for by lay people. Any chiropractors who wanted in just had to form a chapter of PACE. One must understand the historical context of the beginning of PACE to fully appreciate the role it played in chiropractic. At this period the straight chiropractic community was still in its anti-medical mode and PACE was also used as a vehicle to fight against medicine, which was directly and indirectly affecting the advertising and licensing laws. It just so happens that at this particular time, the German measles vaccine was becoming popular and New York's Governor, Nelson Rockefeller, was pushing for a bill to make the measles vaccine mandatory. Sterling Drug Company, manufacturer of the drug and a subsidiary of Standard Oil, a Rockefeller owned company had a campaign going saying "Get under the rubella umbrella (be protected by vaccination)." PACE began to take ads out saying "There's a hole in the rubella umbrella" and gave case histories of children who were crippled after taking the vaccine. The more they ran these ads, the more people would contact PACE with their horror stories of how the drug had injured their child. As a result of PACE many of those children got under chiropractic care and were able to reach more of their potential through regular chiropractic adjustments. The parents became crusaders for PACE. That perhaps best defines PACE. It was a crusade. Parents whose children were harmed by the vaccine had a vehicle to vent their frustrations. Chiropractors had a vehicle to present their approach to health in contrast to the medical approach to disease.

On one occasion PACE took some advertising time on the radio to have testimonials of people injured by the vaccine. Apparently, the programmer did not realize that they were anti-vaccine testimonials and aired them during a program in which a couple of medical doctors were talking about the importance of being vaccinated. Unbeknownst to the MDs and the program host, each time they cut away to a commercial, on would come a PACE ad in which a mother would testify how the vaccine had paralyzed her child or caused arthritis-like problems. I imagine someone got in to a good deal of trouble because of the oversight but it did allow both sides of the story to be told. Irene still laughs twenty-five years later as she relates the story.

The first chapters were formed at one of Reggie's Saturday night philosophy sessions when he presented the idea to the regular attendees. A number of chiropractors signed up their offices at that time. Each chapter had officers made up of the people the chiropractor thought would best help the chapter. The chiropractor would remain the advisor to the chapter. Each chiropractic advisor was given a packet of materials upon the formation of a new chapter. It explained how to organize the chapter, find the right people and begin programs to raise funds for the Association projects. Chapters sprang up in chiropractic offices all over the country as well as in Australia. Of course, there was less attraction in those states that did not have restrictive advertising laws as did New York. Since advertising chiropractic was the main thrust of the organization, this prevented the growth of chapters in those states that had no advertising laws.

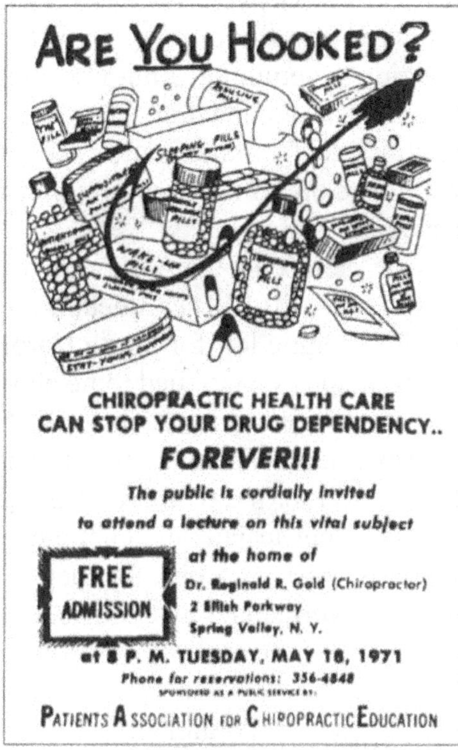

A 1971 newspaper ad sponsored by PACE

PACE was a great practice builder for many chiropractors. It got the patients involved in communicating chiropractic and created a family atmosphere in many offices. Some chapters were barely active at all while others had a tremendous influence in their community. Dr. Jim Doherty's chapter in New Jersey was very active. Dick Plummer was the primary mover in the chapter. He got so much experience communicating chiropractic as a lay person that by the time he was a student at Sherman College he was able to teach the Chiropractic Communications courses at the school. Today, Dick is one of the outstanding communicators in chiropractic and his start came in PACE.

The demise of the ABC was the lack of a strong personality to lead it after Bill Werner's death. PACE too began to wane in activity after Reggie left for South Carolina, although a number of individual chapters continued to be active for a few years. Other factors also contributed to the decline of PACE. Patient organizations seem to be effective when there is a specific issue for them to rally around. During Werner's day, it was the right to chiropractic care. Werner actually went to jail for practicing chiropractic and many patients fervently supported him for that. With PACE, the issue was chiropractic advertising. Once the state laws that prohibited chiropractic advertising were rescinded that motivation was gone. Chiropractors could pay for personal advertising which, although expensive, was much easier than organizing patients to do fund raising.

PACE was able to accomplish a number of things. Some of them we may not consider a priority or even important to straight chiropractic today but at the time, they were perceived as vital. PACE helped influence legislation that created insurance equality for chiropractors. While Reggie and many others had a box on the wall practice, the issue was one of the patient's right to see the doctor of their choice and be covered under their insurance plan. Of course, this was in a time when almost all chiropractors saw chiropractic as an alternative to medicine. Reg had not yet presented chiropractic as a non-duplicating, non-alternative approach to health. One interesting example of the organization's influence occurred in New Jersey. "The Bergen County Record," before PACE, would not even print the word 'chiropractor' because of the income they received in medical advertising. Some years later however, as a result of PACE's persistence, the newspaper ran an editorial in favor of chiropractic having equal representation along with medicine in a governmental agency. PACE helped overcome the restrictive anti-advertising laws in the state of New Jersey where many PACE chapters were located. Health fairs were beginning at malls and at first chiropractic was excluded. PACE picketed these fairs and forced them to include chiropractic. Some local chapters and PACE International also provided some scholarships for Sherman students when the school opened in 1973. Perhaps the most important contribution to chiropractic was the number of chapter officers who ultimately went off to chiropractic college. Three of the four officers of the parent organization PACE International eventually became chiropraetors; Linda Chicarelli, Dick Plummer, and Gerry Giddings all went to Sherman College.

Another factor in the demise of PACE related to the evolution of straight chiropractic. Straight chiropractic as Reggie taught it was getting away from disease. In doing that it became necessary to divorce chiropractic from medical issues. The promiscuous use of drugs, and forced vaccinations, while still important health issues, were no longer relative to straight chiropractic. So PACE, having served its purpose, just sort of faded away.

Whether patient organizations will ever again be effective is an interesting question. There appear to be no issues that affect chiropractors today that are important enough to the lay person to motivate them to carry the chiropractic banner. The anti-medicine attitude of the seventies helped to feed the interest in PACE. The rubella vaccine was being made mandatory in New York and many of the horror stories of its side effects were coming to light. Further, the Wilk case was a few years away so organized medicine was still outwardly antagonistic toward chiropractic. This big bully medicine versus underdog chiropractic attracted many young people who were looking for causes to support. The students who had come through the sixties were still very anti-establishment and there is nothing more establishment then medicine. Chiropractic was anti-drug, appealing to those who had seen the damage of the drug culture and it was in the forefront of the growing interest in "natural living." Chiropractors played on all these factors and it was not difficult to recruit PACE members to go to bat for chiropractic against medicine. Of course, that is not how modern day straight chiropractic is positioning itself. Unless people can be motivated by the importance of getting the life-saving, life-enhancing message of chiropractic out to the world, it is doubtful that lay people can be motivated as a force in chiropractic. That motivation is highly unlikely because most of the chiropractors themselves are not motivated in this area. Further, starting a lay persons organization to help a struggling chiropractor who represents a minority is one thing. Helping a doctor who appears to have equality and is making as much or more than the average medical doctor is something else.

Politics

During this period Reggie was very involved in the political aspect of the chiropractic profession. He was elected to the Representative Assembly of the ICA as the rep from New York State. In the Assembly he was elected Chairman and presided over their annual meetings. It was also during this period that straight chiropractic was beginning to go downhill. A whole new generation of chiropractors who had never been exposed to the philosophy of B.J. were in positions of influence in national and state organizations that had previously been straight. While it would be a few years before the ICA would make the decision to take a seat on the CCE, the handwriting was on the wall. The ICA's accrediting agency was all but an empty shell. Reggie saw this downhill trend and left the ICA, resigning his position as chairman of the Representative Assembly at the same time. Prior to that he had tried to persuade the members of the Representative Assembly of the danger of the direction that the ICA was taking by, among other things, sending the following letter to his fellow RA's:

> Dear Fellow Assemblyman:
>
> I write this letter not as Chairman of your Assembly, but

as a member of it. I am deeply disturbed by the official attitude of ICA towards the subject of differential diagnosis.

If we do not renounce diagnosis entirely as a chiropractic procedure, we face the gravest peril this profession has yet known.

Those who wish to adopt diagnosis put forward several convincing arguments:

1. That it does not belong exclusively to medicine, that it is taught in our schools, that we are examined in it to prove our competence and should protect our right to use it.

2. That the great weapon organized medicine has against us is that too often our failure to properly diagnose prevents us from recognizing those cases that should be referred to other healing arts, thus causing delay in proper medical treatment where needed.

3. That only by using standard diagnostic procedures before and after chiropractic can we compile the necessary research data to prove the efficacy of chiropractic to the scientific and legislative communities.

4. That differential diagnosis is necessary to determine whether any particular patient is a "chiropractic case."

5. That we can't stem the tide of progress.

The fact is that if we do accept diagnosis, we give organized medicine the weapon they need to crucify us.

By our own admission, we would recognize that some diseases are better treated by other healing arts. In accepting this, we concede that we do treat diseases and that whether a patient should be treated by us or by a medical doctor depends upon the nature of the disease and upon its severity.

We must never lose sight of the fact that chiropractors do not treat diseases. Not any diseases. Our practice is limited to the location and correction of vertebral subluxations for the restoration and maintenance of the integrity of the nervous system.

This is necessary for every man, woman and child from the moment of birth to the moment of death, without regard to whatever diseases may or may not be present. The dentist fills cavities, without regard to whether or not the patient has gallstones, ingrown toenails or cancer of the pancreas. We must correct vertebral subluxations with the same impartiality and not get lured into the trap of treating diseases.

If we do treat some diseases and refer others, which do we treat, and which do we refer? Should we take the patient who comes to us after 20 years of ineffective medical treatment for a stomach ulcer, diagnose it as cancer and refer him back to the incompetence of medicine? If trained medical diagnosis is as incompetent as we are told, how accurate can a half-trained diagnosis be? And, make no mistake, all chiropractors are only half-trained in diagnosis. How many cases of Lupus Erythematosis have you seen? How many of Syphilis? Of Lymphatic Leukemia? How often have you been called upon to differentiate between Myasthenia Gravis and Amyotrophic Lateral Sclerosis? Let's face it — the medical doctor learns diagnosis, not from textbooks in school, but upon actual diagnostics, don't be surprised if we are required to intern for one year in a medical hospital-if we can find one to take us.

Furthermore: Diagnosis, even at the hands of the best trained M.D., depends to a large extent on tests not available to a chiropractor. For example, in many states chiropractors are even denied access to lab reports. And what do we think our chances are of getting an angiogram or a pneumoencephalogram or even an electroencephalogram on a patient? And, if we refer him to an M.D. for the test, we'll never see him again. In either case, are these tests chiropractically desirable?

Imagine yourself in the witness chair. "Would you attempt chiropractic on a herniated disc?" "No?" How would you know whether any low back case is a herniated disc or not when the only recognized diagnostic test for a herniated disc is a myelogram? No chiropractor worthy of the name would allow his worst enemy to undergo such butchery as a myelogram.

If the question of whether a case is for chiropractic or for referral to medicine is to be determined by differential diagnosis, obviously it should happen after a truly competent diagnostician (M.D.) has determined that that is what is indicated. Get the point????????? Since the MD's are the only competent diagnosticians, and the only ones with access to all diagnostic procedures, they and not us are the logical ones to determine which therapy is indicated in any given case.

If chiropractic is to survive, we must renounce all claims to diagnose, stop becoming medical referral centers and get back to the principle that only a spinal analysis can determine whether or not anyone is a chiropractic case. If there is subluxation, he is. If not, he is not.

As far as proof to the scientific and legislative communities is concerned, their expert authority on all matters of health is the medical profession. We furnish clinical proof which is then turned over to medical experts for unbiased evaluation. Nuf said? Besides research data, if it is to be valid, it must be done under controlled conditions by a chiropractic research team not by the practicing chiropractor in his office. Another excuse shot down.

For years now we have allowed weakness and compromise to steadily chip away at the philosophical heart of chiropractic. The so-called "Chicago definition" gave open sesame to all kinds of mixing done as "procedures preparatory to and complimentary to" the chiropractic adjustment and "the establishment of patient regimen" from the same definition is a sop to the vitamin peddlers in our ranks.

We are told we must learn to compromise. But compromise means we must give up something in order to receive something else in return. What were we given in return for the straight definition we gave away? Was it ours to give away in the first place?

Step by step we have reduced chiropractic until it is fast becoming spinal manipulation for the relief of neuro-musculo-skeletal symptoms without any other purpose or philosophy.

That is the thinking of the so-called "Liberal" in chiropractic. It is not and must never become the thinking of ICA. ICA exists to nurture and protect chiropractors. As B.J. said, "It is taking the line of least resistance that makes rivers and men crooked." We must not only hold the line against the encroachment of compromised political thinking-we must actually take back that part of our principle that we have been giving away. If we don't do that, ICA is finished. Spinal therapy will survive for another decade or so and then that, too, will be taken over and swallowed up by medicine.

I write to you assemblymen about this because I want your active support. Please contact your constituents and see if they share my views and then write and let me know the consensus of field opinion. Your wishes and your constituents' wishes must formulate the policy of ICA If you don't participate in this survey,

I must assume you don't care one way of the other.

Please answer me. Not a long letter. Just a note to say whether you and yours support my viewpoint or the liberal viewpoint.

Yours very truly,

Reginald R. Gold, D.C., Ph.C.
Chairman of Representative Assembly

Distribution: All ICA Representative Assemblymen

Copies to: All Executive Officers
Board of Control Members
Heads of ICA Colleges
Legal Council
Executive Director

Reg's letter fell on deaf ears. Actually, the Representative Assembly were by and large straight but the Board of Control, the real power in the ICA, was committed to a more therapeutic approach to chiropractic. However, during that time in the ICA, Reggie met another Palmer graduate who was the assemblyman from South Carolina. His name was Thomas A. Gelardi.

Reggie could see the direction of the chiropractic profession moving in a more therapeutic direction. There were more mixers, more modalities and so-called straights were getting into nutrition and rehabilitation exercises. Reggie was not trying to hold the line against this drift toward medicine, he was actually trying to take chiropractic in the opposite direction. There were (and still are) three distinct schools of thought in chiropractic. The first would like to see chiropractic move in the direction of medicine and become like the osteopathic profession. Within that group are the disease treaters who argue over whether or not to use drugs. The second group are those who want chiropractic to remain as in B.J.'s day. They address diseases and their cause. Most of them want to correct subluxations only, but they agree to the need for diagnosis to determine whether limitations of matter have been exceeded and referral is necessary. The third group of which Reggie is the most articulate spokesman, wants to move chiropractic away from the disease model and toward enhancing potential in all areas of life.

Even in the early seventies, the lines between the three groups were becoming more clearly defined. It was clear to Reg that the first group represented nothing that resembled the chiropractic of B.J. The second group was clearly an impractical position, trying to sit on the straight chiropractic fence, but caving in to the demands of an increasingly medicalized profession. Reggie had decided that the colleges were all going in the wrong direction, the "ACA schools" by intent, the "ICA schools," including his alma mater Palmer, by default. He had also decided to move his practice, which had outgrown the 2 Ellish Parkway location to another part of town. Reggie also planned to start a post-graduate chiropractic school, where chiropractors could enroll for a three-month period and learn how to practice a non-therapeutic type of chiropractic, and important aspects of patient education that earmarked his practice and were responsible for its phenomenal growth. They would also learn adjusting technique because these programs at chiropractic colleges were suffering as a result of the increased diagnostic course material. He bought a piece of ground on South Main Street in Spring Valley and hired an architect to design the facility. Then a call came from South Carolina from Thom Gelardi, telling Reggie of his plans to begin a new chiropractic college, the first one in almost twenty-five years.

CHAPTER 3

The South Carolina Experience

1972-1977

Dr. Thom Gelardi of Gaffney, South Carolina decided to start a new chiropractic college. He elicited the help of another area chiropractor, Dr. Michael Kale from nearby Spartanburg. There is some difference of opinion over the purpose of the new school. Gelardi maintains that it was to preserve straight chiropractic, given the direction the ICA and the "ICA schools" were going, and in the opinion of many, it ultimately served that purpose. Reggie and others say that it was primarily to preserve the HIO technique of B.J. which Palmer College was quickly abandoning. It was hard enough to keep chiropractors on the spine, let alone on one or two bones. The fact that both Gelardi and Kale were committed to Upper Cervical Specific would support Reggie's contention (and the understanding of the chiropractors whose memories go back that far, myself included). It would also seem reasonable that two largely unknown chiropractors (in 1972), who wanted to begin a school based upon a quickly dying but very important and valuable technique would want a national figure to help draw students and professional support. Whatever the case, they asked Reggie to come to the school. Reggie made it clear that as a full spine practitioner, he had no interest in promoting HIO but he did have a tremendous desire and passion to teach and promulgate his "non-therapeutic" approach to chiropractic. It is fortunate for Sherman that someone as popular and well-known as Reggie was a full-spine practitioner. For in the first few years of Sherman, the heavy emphasis upon HIO created concern among field chiropractors. Many times Reggie had to placate a straight, full-spine chiropractor in the field who had sent a student to Sherman only to have the student return home on break and" inform his chiropractor that he was a mixer because he adjusted below Axis. As a representative of Sherman, Reggie was able to satisfy these Sherman supporters that was not the position of the school.

The school was to be named after Lyle W. Sherman, who was a former director of the B.J. Palmer Chiropractic Clinic in Davenport and to whom Dr. Gelardi owed the restoration of his health. By the early seventies, Palmer College had all but abandoned upper cervical technique, especially the knee-chest adjustment that Dr. Sherman used. Ironically, Palmer began teaching full spine for the first time to Reggie's class.

But the teaching was done with very little enthusiasm and the emphasis was still on HIO. "We were taught full-spine but also taught to sneer at it," Reg recalls. When he graduated he considered himself a full-spine practitioner but admits he was not terribly proficient at it. Dr. Pepper and other chiropractors gave him help. That is one reason why Reggie has always had such an interest in specific, gentle, full-spine work.

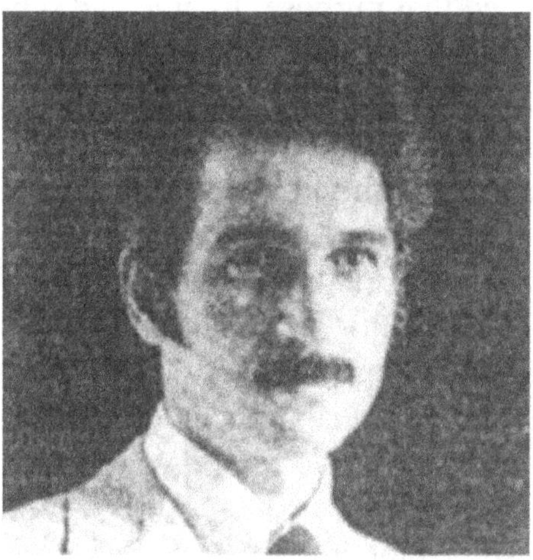

Thomas A. Gelardi, D.C. Founder and president of Sherman College of Straight Chiropractic

Sixteen years later, after full spine technique was first taught, it had taken over the technique curriculum. Whether the formation of Sherman was to preserve the upper cervical technique as Reg and others maintain or not, in no way lessens the importance of what Thom Gelardi did in starting the school. The entire straight chiropractic community owes a debt of gratitude to the man for his vision and perseverance in founding and developing Sherman College. Reggie himself makes it clear that it was Thom's idea and Thom's school from the start. He maintains that, "Thom is a strong and capable leader." Reggie was happy to serve under him and to help build the philosophy of the school while he recognized that Thom was ultimately responsible for Sherman's direction.

At this time, the chiropractic profession, including the straight schools were in a head-long rush toward medicalization. The mixing schools had always been moving in that direction, but now the ICA schools were jumping on the band wagon. Coming to a clinical impression, which included a medical diagnosis, had never been an issue to the straight schools. Monitoring of medical conditions by straight chiropractors was only done to determine that the body was healing itself of a medical condition that had previously been diagnosed and unsuccessfully treated by a physician. The straight chiropractors who did medical tests only did so to demonstrate that they and chiropractic were getting the sick person well where medicine had failed. It was never for the purpose of referral or to determine the need for therapeutic interventions. However, this position was tenuous at best from a legal malpractice stand point and confusing to the public which was becoming more and more disease oriented and medically astute. People were also starting to go to chiropractors first and so if a chiropractor was going to address a medical condition or its cause, a diagnosis needed to be made to insure that the chiropractor could expect to get the sick person well and crisis medical intervention was not necessary. Reg felt that the only way to stop this medicalization of chiropractic was to present chiropractors in a totally non-therapeutic light. The idea was to present chiropractic as the correction of vertebral subluxation alone because, as he so concisely put it in his letter to the Representative Assembly years before, "This is necessary for every man, woman and child from the moment of birth to the moment of death, without regard to whatever diseases may or may not be present." With this model of chiropractic, the diagnosis of medical conditions was not necessary, in fact, it was counter productive to the patient's understanding. Without the need for a medical diagnosis, there was no need for medical tests, physical examinations, laboratory tests, diagnostic x-rays and the myriad of other procedures normally associated with medical practice that were quickly being appropriated by the chiropractic profession. It was only necessary for the chiropractor to locate, analyze and correct vertebral subluxations and of course communicate to the patient the uniqueness and singularity of the chiropractic objective.

Reggie did not care which methods and techniques for locating and correcting subluxations were used as long as they did what they were suppose to do and had a philosophical basis. He did, however, have some strong ideas about how to teach the philosophy. Further, he had some new and unique ideas about communicating chiropractic to the public and making the chiropractic college graduate competent in that endeavor. By now he had done thousands of lay lectures, radio and television shows, and one on one orientations and he was anxious to share the techniques associated with these important educational endeavors with students so they in turn could build large practices, full of patients getting adjusted for the right reason. He saw the college as an opportunity to teach some new and innovative approaches to patient education. The ideas that he had hoped to put into the post-graduate program in Spring Valley could be taught to students in chiropractic college so that the day they graduated from Sherman, they would be prepared to do a lay lecture, to answer patient's questions in a philosophically correct manner and to communicate chiropractic to the lay and medical community.

Reggie sold his home in Spring Valley to Ernie Landi and turned his patients over to him. At the time, Irene was in her last year at Columbia, by this time known as New York Chiropractic College. She had decided to enroll there because of the close proximity to the Spring Valley home. Since Sherman was beginning with a freshman class, it would have been impossible for her to transfer to Sherman unless she wanted to take a leave of her chiropractic education for two years until Sherman's freshman class caught up with her. They decided that she should finish up at the New York school and Reggie would head south to help develop the college in Spartanburg.

Reg threw himself into Sherman. He was involved in every aspect of the school, from cutting and pasting catalogs from other chiropractic colleges to form Sherman's on the living room floor of Thom's house to traveling all over the country recruiting. He and Thom worked side by side, beginning what would be a lifelong friendship between the two men. As with any new school, faculty and administrators find themselves teaching anything and everything. In the beginning, Reg taught Philosophy, Terminology, and Technique. But his main passion was teaching communications. Palmer had a public speaking course but it did not teach the student how to communicate chiropractic. No one had ever taken the chiropractic philosophy and distilled it into a simple message that could be understood by the average lay person. Stephenson's *Chiropractic Textbook* was hard enough for students to read for an understanding the philosophy. It was an insurmountable task for lay people. But Reggie made the philosophy simple, logical and exciting. He taught it to students and taught them how to teach it.

Reggie had to adapt a number of his courses from Columbia to develop a philosophy curriculum for Sherman. Unlike the science courses and "medical courses" that could be adopted from the soon to be CCE schools, no one had a true philosophy course. Palmer set aside the B.J. philosophy (as presented in Stephenson's textbook) after Galen Price left the Philosophy department. He was replaced by Dr. Virgil Strang who is currently the President of Palmer College. Strang had written his own philosophy text which was a collection of scientific and eclectic musings. Despite the fact that the book gets mixed reviews, it became the required text for the course and the course was built around it. Whether it is good or bad, one thing is for sure, it is not a deductive systematic approach to explaining the chiropractic philosophy. If the big idea is found in it, it is not evident, especially to a first quarter student. So Reggie and Thom worked closely together to develop a philosophy curriculum for Sherman.

While they had some help with the philosophy courses namely,

Stephenson, Price's philosophy course that both Reggie and Thom had taken and Reggie's curriculum from Columbia, they had nothing with respect to a Communication course. That would be one of the hallmarks of the new college. Communication was going to be a large part of the philosophy curriculum. As Reggie puts it, "Teaching philosophy as an abstract subject is almost valueless. You have to be able to pass it on to other people. It is a wonderful basis for your own life but beyond that, to be of service to the community you have to simplify it. My forte has always been the ability to simplify it and then to teach the technique of getting it across to the public."

Since there was no established curriculum, Reggie developed it as he went along. He was without doubt the most qualified person in the world to develop a Communication curriculum. He had given more lay lectures, answered more patient questions and explained the philosophy to more lay people than any other chiropractor alive. He had done hundreds of radio shows and been in dozens of debates. Verbal communication was the hallmark of the Communication course and it evolved as they went along. Sherman students were fortunate to have Reg initiate this and also fortunate to have other chiropractors like Joe Flesia, Guy Riekman and Doug Gates join the faculty and continue to develop and expand the Philosophy and the Communication programs. Dick Plummer, as a student at Sherman, having come from Jim Doherty's office, without doubt contributed as much as anyone to the development of the communication curriculum and even today, over twenty years since the beginning of the school, Plummer's influence can be seen in Sherman's communication curriculum.

There had not been a new chiropractic college in nearly twenty-five years. They had to model their curriculum after the established schools to meet state laws and soon-to-be-established accrediting standards. Yet they also had different ideas about what chiropractic was, what constituted a chiropractic education and, most important, what philosophy they would be teaching. In addition to the differences between Sherman and the other schools, there were also differences among the supporters of the school. The non-therapeutic approach that Reggie was developing in his mind was foreign even to the average 1972 straight chiropractor. Other than a few people who had regular exposure to Reggie in Spring Valley, very few had already grasped the big idea of non-diagnostic, non-therapeutic, straight chiropractic. It was not unheard of for a straight chiropractor to wear a white lab coat, to have a functional stethoscope and sphygmomanometer sitting on his desk or to talk about subluxation as the cause of the patient's medical problem. The diagnosis issue which would eventually be the focal point of argument was yet to be clearly defined. No one in the chiropractic profession was in any way competent in the area of diagnosis. The straights of the day did not pretend to be, although usually they made some attempt at telling the patient what medical problem they had. Chiropractic had been a "last resort," so historically most patients had already been previously diagnosed. The reason that diagnosis became the defining argument between Reggie's and Sherman's non-therapeutic approach and all other approaches (traditional straight and all degrees of mixing) was that diagnosis is the necessary starting point for a therapeutic approach. If you choose not to make a medical diagnosis, you are in fact saying that your procedure is of a non-therapeutic nature. Conversely, if you choose to diagnose you are implying a therapeutic procedure and it is incumbent upon you that you have a degree of expertise in that area. This was truly the defining point in the chiropractic profession. It was at this point that part of the profession, those practicing the objective straight approach espoused by Reggie, deliberately moved away from the therapeutic model. The rest of the profession moved toward the therapeutic approach whether consciously or unconsciously as did the traditional straight chiropractors with the idea of getting sick people well. One way or the other, diagnosis was a stumbling block.

This was the setting in which Sherman opened in 1972. Consequently, Reggie saw the importance of first getting this idea across to those associated with Sherman and then to students coming from field practitioners who likely did not have this vision of straight chiropractic. Thom Gelardi was amenable to what Reggie wanted to do and Sherman College of Chiropractic threw its energies into not only preserving Upper Cervical technique but to teaching this visionary approach to straight chiropractic to both students and the profession.

Reggie as a teacher was Reggie in every other way. He was either loved by his students or he was hated by them. There was no middle ground as far as the students' attitude toward him was concerned. Simply because there was no middle ground for Reg. He took chiropractic philosophy and the teaching of it very seriously. When he began his class, he locked his door and those that were not there on time missed the class. Students who were lackadaisical about chiropractic philosophy did not like this policy. Those that were committed did not want to miss a word of his lecture. From Reggie's standpoint, it was not a matter of being unyielding or petty. He contends that having people walk in late for class disrupts the concentration of the teacher and the other students and may cause those that were conscientious enough to get there on time to miss an important point. The tone for the entire lecture might be set in the first few minutes. A late student might well miss an important concept and often ended up asking unnecessary questions. Not to mention it is rude, inconsiderate and demonstrates a lack of self discipline to be late. Reggie's feeling was if people did not have good manners and self-discipline by the time they entered chiropractic college, it was time to learn them. Late students were able to hear the lecture from the hallway and on more than one occasion students could be seen sitting on the floor next to the doorway while Reg was in the classroom lecturing.

In the first quarter, students were not allowed to ask questions until he completed the subject matter. If it took an entire class to develop a concept, they may not even get to ask a question that day. Reggie was adamant about students challenging the philosophy before they had a semester's foundation. A man who was adept at answering challenges from some of the sharpest medical and mixer-chiropractic minds in the country was not afraid of a first semester student. But he disliked answering questions that would be able to be answered by the student himself or herself with another hour or two of philosophy. Reggie felt that teaching students to think for themselves and logically deduce the answers to questions was the greatest knowledge he could impart to the student. Standing up in front of a class, fielding question after question, is impressive to a freshman student but teaching them to think from an above down-inside out perspective was much more important and what he strived for in the classroom. Students who did not want to think for themselves or were lazy often walked away from a class frustrated because he would not take questions. They were the ones who did not like Reggie. Those that accepted his challenge to think are some of the great minds in straight chiropractic today. Reggie taught the students what the chiropractors and others were learning on Saturday nights in Spring Valley. There was not much difference between Reggie who lectured in New York and the Reggie who taught the students in South Carolina. Reggie was Reggie. He never tried to be anybody or anything else. On the contrary, the focus was always on what he was teaching and the beauty and simplicity of the chiropractic philosophy, never on the man himself. His delivery, as powerful as it was, always focused on the message not on the messenger. And his delivery was superb. He was entertaining, often humorous, yet he could tug at your heart strings, create emotion, inspire and motivate you. Somehow, it never seemed like it was those things that got to you. It always seemed it was chiropractic. With some chiropractic speakers, you get the feeling that they could substitute Amway or anything else for chiropractic and deliver the same message in the same way. With Reggie, you get the feeling that if he were talking about anything but chiropractic he would not be as captivating a speaker.

The outstanding outcome of Reggie's teaching days at Sherman has to be the systematization of the straight chiropractic philosophy. Until Reggie went to Sherman, the chiropractic philosophy was not being taught anywhere in a systematic manner. In fact, it was not being taught at all at most chiropractic colleges. As mentioned earlier, some philosophy was being taught at Palmer, but the course really only presented a fragment of the systematic philosophy as Galen Price had tried to teach it. Many schools taught "Chiropractic Principles," usually as an historic aspect of our profession, like Harvey Lillard's deafness. Some, like Strang and Dr. Frank Digiacamo at NYCC, were teaching their textbooks which were bits and pieces of the philosophy. Even Reg, prior to going to Sherman, was only delivering a smattering of the philosophy because almost every time he spoke it was to a different audience. Even the Saturday night sessions drew a constant influx of new people who needed to hear the basics. Sherman represented an opportunity for Reg to present the philosophy in a logical, deductive manner, building upon a foundation and taking the student to a deep and lasting understanding. It is true Reg had taught at Columbia into the mid-sixties, but by 1973 he had developed the non-therapeutic approach to chiropractic. Sherman gave him the opportunity to teach it in a 60-hour module.

B.J. wrote a book entitled *Conflicts Clarify.* There is probably no conflict in modern-day chiropractic that has done more to clarify the straight chiropractic philosophy than the issue of diagnosis. Reggie, understandably, has been the focal point of this issue. Sherman, its philosophy and the advent of the CCE during the colleges early development pitted the non-diagnostic and the diagnostic approaches against one another. Reggie realized, and worked toward making the straight chiropractic community aware that this was the issue that would ultimately determine whether one had a chiropractic objective or a medical objective. If your objective is truly chiropractic, to correct subluxations for better expression of the innate intelligence, then diagnosis is not only not called for, it is contradicted for it creates confusion in the patient's mind as to what your objective is. This necessitated some "fine tuning to clarify" the chiropractic philosophy, something Reggie had already done but something most of the straight community had not yet accomplished and that many of them were opposed to doing for one reason or another. This conflict divided the straight chiropractic community into what has come to be known as the traditional straights and the objective straights of whom Reggie was the most articulate spokesperson.

Surprisingly, diagnosis had never been a major issue in the chiropractic profession. It was one of those subjects in chiropractic that no one discussed or made an issue of, almost as if no one ever thought about it. It took someone like Reg to articulate that diagnosis was totally inconsistent with the chiropractic objective. If chiropractic was not an alternative to or a substitute for medicine then it was not necessary to diagnose. If the chiropractor was correcting a cause of DIS-EASE (lack of innate expression) and not the cause of disease (medical entities) then diagnosis was not necessary. Coincidental with the development of logical deduction as it applies to chiropractic philosophy that Reggie began teaching at Sherman, was a marked interest in incorporating diagnosis and even expanding its usage in the practice of chiropractic by other members of the profession. As mentioned earlier, since the chiropractor had previously been seen as a last resort, the need for him to diagnose was a moot point. People going to the chiropractor had already received a medical diagnosis (and usually treatment which had failed). For the chiropractor to diagnose the same condition when he was going to try something different (correcting subluxations) was a waste of time. At this time, however, chiropractors were beginning to see people who had not seen any other doctor, although mostly for musculoskeletal problems. They were also beginning to fill out medical insurance forms that required a "diagnosis." The medically oriented insurance companies were an ideal pawn for the diagnosing segment of the profession. Further, seeing patients for the treatment, cure or prevention of medical problems by non-medical means necessitated diagnostic skills on the part of the chiropractor and it was clear to all segments of the profession that the average chiropractic student's level of expertise was woefully low. The mixing aspect of the profession was more than happy to try to raise that level and since they controlled the accreditation process for the profession, they coerced the traditional straights into agreeing to the need for diagnosis in chiropractic education and practice. Although they tried to justify it with the traditional straight chiropractic philosophy set down by B.J., to which they claimed to subscribe, it obviously cannot be justified in any rational way. Reggie has a unique ability to explain the logical, rational, deductive basis for what had become his approach to straight chiropractic. In doing so, he began to point out the irrationality of the traditional approach as practiced by Palmer, Logan, the Clevelands and the ICA. The traditional straights were in a delicate position. They had one foot in philosophical chiropractic as a result of their reverence for D.D. and B.J. and one foot in medical chiropractic, a position they were forced to remain in as a result of the CCE's control over them. The more Reggie pointed out the fallacy of their position, the more the above organizations rebelled and tried to attack and denigrate the man and his approach. He was not allowed on the campus of some schools which claimed to be straight. Nevertheless, hundreds of students saw the philosophical, rational and practical reasons for practicing the objective straight chiropractic that Reggie was teaching, off campus at these schools and on campus at Sherman.

From this point, straight chiropractic course material began to be taught, not from the standpoint of an alternative to medicine or of a drugless healing art, but from a position of whether the subject matter helped to achieve the chiropractic objective or not. Clearly, from this perspective, diagnosis was totally unacceptable as part of the education of the student and part of the practice of the chiropractor. The mixing portion of the profession was focusing their energies almost entirely on diagnosis. They recognized that it was the one thing the medical profession could legitimately criticize that chiropractors could not and did not do adequately, in practice. Of course, the mixing portion of the profession had long ago given up the nerve interference idea and the concept that an adjustment enables the body's inborn wisdom to be more fully expressed. They apparently saw themselves as treaters of muscoskeletal problems and referral doctors for the medical physician. It was about this time the federal government was becoming more and more involved in health care delivery and developed the term Primary Health Care Provider (PHCP). To the mixers, this was a godsend. If chiropractors were PHCPs then they finally had parity with the medical doctor which was the ultimate goal of most of the mixing aspect of the profession, to be "real doctors." This term was also just what the traditional straights were looking for. Many of them realized that there was no logical or rational reason to be diagnosing and that it was inconsistent with the chiropractic philosophy of

B. J. which they still held to. They felt that their behavior was excusable now that the federal government had given them a title which necessitates that they diagnose. Their reasoning was that in order to determine whether chiropractic adjustments could enable the body to heal itself or not, the chiropractor must first determine what the condition was. (Author's Note: No one has any idea whether the body has passed its limitations of matter or not. Every chiropractor has seen dozens of supposedly incurable people get better and people with apparently minor problems get no better or actually get worse under chiropractic care. So even from the traditional "chiropractic gets sick people well" standpoint, diagnosis and prognosis is impossible. That is why traditional straight chiropractic is an untenable position.)

Fortunately, by the time the term Primary Health Care Provider had been created by the government, Reggie had already perfectly positioned straight chiropractic to be able to avoid the diagnosis issue. If chiropractic was not addressing medical conditions or their cause , then diagnosis was not necessary. The chiropractor could still be a PHCP with the straight model and argue very logically for that position. A PHCP was merely a provider that the public could go to first, without need for a referral from another health care provider. Objective straight chiropractic fit perfectly into that description in as far as there is no one able to determine whether a person needs chiropractic care or not except a chiropractor. Of course the logical conclusion is that the only person who can properly determine whether someone needs medical care or not is a medical doctor. Following this line of reasoning eliminates the need for medical diagnosis by chiropractors, to the dismay of mixers. It also eliminates the potential for chiropractors to tell a patient when and if they needed medical care, to the dismay of the traditional straights. Unfortunately, the traditional straights could not abandon their anti-medical position. They wanted the opportunity to tell people that they no longer needed medical care or that chiropractors could "fix" their medical problems or their causes. They hid this desire in statements like "Being responsible as a doctor." But the term "doctor" is such a nebulous term, that it was really a smoke screen for their "medical alternative" brand of chiropractic. As vice president of Sherman College in January 1976, Reg wrote a letter to David A. Kindig, M.D., Deputy Director of the Department of Health Education and Welfare requesting a clarification of the term Primary Health Care Provider. He received a letter from Dr. Kindig's response. The letter said in part,

> "...there is no intent or authorization to change or even define the authority, scope of practice or function of the occupation concerned. Therefore, the term 'Primary Health Care Provider' as it is applied to chiropractors has no effect upon statutes and regulations which define or limit the scope of chiropractic, and does not permit them to perform diagnostic examinations of the entire body. Similarly, this term does not mandate chiropractors to perform diagnostic examinations of the entire body."

The first five years of Sherman College were perhaps the most important period in straight chiropractic history. The school was creating and developing a straight chiropractic curriculum. The focus was upon Philosophy. While the subjects being taught were essentially the same as at other schools, they were being taught from a straight perspective. Most of the chiropractic colleges were moving toward having Ph.D.s teach their basic science courses. Regardless of whether the professor was a vitalist or not. Sherman, on the other hand, wanted assurance that all of the faculty accepted the vitalistic philosophy of straight chiropractic. What was being taught by every faculty member had to agree with objective straight chiropractic. This was unique to chiropractic colleges.

Many of the Ph.D.s teaching at Sherman ended up becoming students there and eventually chiropractors, something virtually unheard of at other chiropractic colleges. This attests to the attractiveness of the objective straight philosophy to intelligent, scientific minds and to the ability of Thom Gelardi to choose people who would be so interested in the philosophy that they would want to become chiropractors and practice it themselves.

Not only was the faculty at Sherman College unique, but the students were also a special group of people, perhaps unlike any other group of students in the history of the profession. The first several classes came to a new school with no accreditation and an accrediting agency (CCE) that did not reflect or support their philosophy. They could have gone to other schools which were well established and possibly closer to their homes. Interestingly, students came to ADIO Institute under the same circumstances six years later but most of them were attracted by the convenience of the location. While many students went to schools in the 20's and 30's knowing it was illegal to practice in their home state, they knew that every other student at every other school was in the same position. The Sherman students knew there was a chance they would not be allowed to practice simply because of where they were educated. And they still chose to go there. They did so to learn a philosophy that they believed was more important than where they could set up practice. Many of them were never able to return to their home states to practice. Some of the students went to Sherman because they had heard Reggie talk, but most of the students were sent to Sherman by their field chiropractors because *they* had heard Reggie talk. Either way. Reggie's ability to attract students to Sherman was undeniable. In addition, it was the early seventies. There were still many who had the idealism of the sixties who had heard the words of John Kennedy when he said, " Ask not what your country can do for you, but what you can do for your country." There were those who had challenged the authority of the government over Vietnam and many were still in the rebel mode. "Us against the world," both the medical world and the greater part of the chiropractic world, drew the students and faculty together as a tightly knit group of chiropractic revolutionaries. Reggie was their leader. Using his extraordinary communication skills, he taught a model of chiropractic that was revolutionary even to those that followed B.J. Some became known as "Reggie's Raiders," a term which was first used in derision but eventually became a badge of honor. Thom and Reggie formed a unique balance. Thom projected the establishment, conservative image that was necessary to deal with the rest of the chiropractic profession and Reggie created the enthusiasm and fervor that kept the students fired up. Thom handled business with government agencies and day-to-day administrative responsibilities while Reg constantly worked to build and reinforce the students' understanding of the philosophy. Thom wore the three piece suit and Reggie wore the wild clothes. The profession could identify with Gelardi, the students with Gold. Thom dealt with the alligators and Reggie was there to remind everybody that their objective was to drain the swamp. While Thom was in complete control of the school, he recognized Reggie as a most valuable asset and rarely questioned him. As a result of their combined talents and efforts, Sherman grew.

Unfortunately, the accreditation issue hung over Sherman's head despite the school's growth. By 1975, all of the chiropractic schools in the country had capitulated to the pressure of CCE and all were justifying their association with CCE, as the late Dr. Mazzarelli, ICA President put it, because they "were the only game in town." This was true, only because the traditional straight community, especially the ICA, had let the "other game" be run out of town. Thom, concerned about the students being able to go back to their home states and more states opening to Sherman, made the decision to seek CCE accreditation. Reggie recollects that he did not know of the decision and would have opposed it. The CCE in the mid-seventies was a far cry from the CCE of today. The CCE today is made up primarily of educators. Twenty-five years ago, it was largely chiropractors and with few exceptions, ACA-type chiropractors and active, political types at that. Despite this, Thom believed that Sherman could get a fair evaluation from the CCE, after all, an accrediting agency

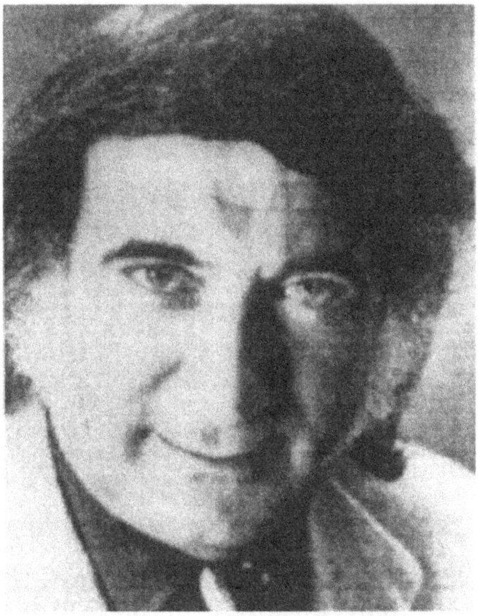

as pictured in the 1973 PACE Testimonial and Farewell Dinner Program

is supposed to be non-political. Accrediting agencies are not intended to judge the merits of a school's philosophy or objective or in the case of religious schools, their theology. They are just supposed to determine whether they are doing a good job in teaching it. The CCE had another agenda. Sherman as pictured in the 1973 PACE failed the inspection and was denied accreditation based on their educational program. It was clear to everyone that the denial had nothing to do with the quality of the education but with the objective of the education. Sherman's education prepared the students for straight chiropractic practice. The CCE felt that it did not prepare the students for their idea of what a chiropractor should do. As a result of this denial, many states that had been opened to Sherman graduates, closed. While there wasn't panic, there was concern, along with a decrease in enrollment and an increase in transfers.

Sherman was anxious to be approved by the South Carolina State Board so that, if nothing else, locals could be attracted to the school and good chiropractors could stay on as faculty as well as practice. Thom was informed that as long as Reggie was associated with Sherman, the College would never be approved by the South Carolina Board. At that time the State board was controlled by members of the South Carolina Chiropractic Association which was antagonistic toward the school. Michael Kale who had been with the school at its formation was influential in the state, and at this time vehemently opposed both the school and Reggie. Kale was a member of the South Carolina Board at that time and was in a position to affect Sherman's approval. Reggie agreed to step down and disassociate himself from the school. It came as a shock to the student body as well as many supporters around the country. In fact, some students tried to mount a campaign to have him reinstated. However, Reg was in agreement with Thom that his departure was necessary. The other concern was whether Sherman could survive without the man who unquestionably was the major attraction for the students, the major fund raiser for the college and the heart and soul of the philosophy department. While it sent shock waves around the straight chiropractic community and shook the school, the person who seemed to be affected the least by it was Reggie. Reg does not live his life with long-term goals in mind. He lives from day-to-day just doing what needs to be done at the time. He had never envisioned himself making a long-term commitment to Sherman, although he had no intention of leaving at that time. But to say he experienced no pain in leaving would deny the love and commitment of the man to the college and the special place in his heart and soul that Sherman College of Straight Chiropractic has. He had given up his practice for Sherman. He had turned his back on his national organization and had spoken out against the things that were going on at Palmer, his alma mater. Sherman College was his home, was the one place on the earth that he identified with and which now closely identifies with his philosophy. To say that there was no feeling of pain and loss at leaving would deny the humanity of the man.

Reggie left Sherman and immediately launched into his next project, the formation of the Federation of Straight Chiropractic Organizations (FSCO). Irene was still teaching at Sherman so it would have been impossible for Reg to leave the area without again separating from her. Besides, he had no particular place to go and what he was now embarking upon could be done from ADIO Flouse, the name of his home in the Spartanburg area. ADIO Flouse was a large ranch style home surrounded by acres of wooded area. It was situated just off of Main Street in Spartanburg. From his home he could put together the Constitution and By-Laws of the FSCO and use

South Carolina as a base for doing seminars and lectures. Reggie did not become a stranger to the school. Students had a standing invitation to his swimming pool Mondays, Wednesdays and Fridays. The basement of ADIO House was a lecture room covered with epigrams where students met once a month for philosophy sessions with Reg. He would often come to address a class or the student body and could regularly be seen in the coffee shop next to the school talking to the students, where he also sharpened his pinball playing skills. Reg could be seen riding around town on his moped during this time, but he was anything but idle. The idea of a new national organization had been simmering in his mind and that of others. With the ICA schools joining the CCE, the ICA was no longer a force in the accreditation field. Their accrediting agency, the ACC, was all but defunct. The ICA itself was making overtures to the CCE and by 1976 would assume a seat on the CCE board. Besides the obvious accreditation issue, it was clear that the ICA was no longer representing the straight community and had drifted from the philosophy of B.J. While Reggie and the objective straights were moving further and further away from a disease model of chiropractic, the ICA was moving closer, so close that they could one day come within a few votes of merging with the ACA. It was not only that they were not representing the objective straights, but many of the leaders in the ICA were mixing, that is, using modalities and/or treating disease. It was clear also that Sid Williams' master plan included taking over the ICA. His D.E. movement was a powerful force and provided the financial base for the support of his new school, Life Chiropractic College. Life College had begun with twenty-two students, but by this time was growing so rapidly that it could well become the largest chiropractic college in the country, something Sid had no reservation in boasting as his goal. There was no longer any relationship between Sid and Reggie or Sid and Thom Gelardi as the respective schools moved in different directions. All of these events and circumstances indicated that there was a need for an organization that would represent the philosophy of Reggie, Sherman College and the straight chiropractic community.

Reggie sat by his pool on those sunny, summer days working on the details of the FSCO. He was determined that the organization be put together as tightly as possible to ensure its success. While the straight community was more in agreement as to what chiropractic was than the ICA or ACA, there were still divergent opinions that had to be considered without compromising the philosophy which had become more and more specific. There was a strong upper cervical group that despite their overt tolerance of full spine adjusters, deep down believed that subluxation did not occur below axis. There were also those who used adjusting instruments, who had previously been on the fringe of straight chiropractic because of the traditional definition of B.J. that said "by hand only." There was a small but vocal group that still held to a "hands only" philosophy. They felt that B.J. had used that term for a specific reason and that hand held adjusting instruments were not straight chiropractic. In addition to these factions, there were the usual political and personality problems to deal with. Putting together an organization for chiropractors, especially ones who strongly held to an uncompromising philosophy was no easy task. Reg wanted to be sure that he had covered all the bases before getting a group of straight chiropractors together. He knew that the slightest difference might trigger a disagreement so terrible that it would destroy the possibility of getting the organization off the ground. He wanted to have the organizational structure well thought out and the Constitution and By-Laws prepared for the meeting. On the other hand, he knew that chiropractors might balk if they thought that something was being forced on them. To find the balance was the key.

Apparently Reg was able to find that balance. Because in August 1976, a group of chiropractors met together in the Clayton House Hotel in Davenport, Iowa to form the Federation of Straight Chiropractic Organizations. Some in attendance had come to Davenport specifically for the meeting. There were also chiropractors there for the ICA Convention and Representative Assembly meetings. Some students like Dick Plummer, Mark Peters, Walt Giddings and Ken Hillman had even come from Spartanburg. Reg chaired the meeting and the Constitution and By-Laws were discussed and ratified as was the definition of chiropractic. This significant event may very well have been the re-defining of chiropractic. While many in the group were B.J. people and resisted changing the definition, the ICA had already created a new definition a few years before adding the "preparatory to" phrase which had opened the door for modalities. The uniqueness of the FSCO definition was that it clearly defined chiropractic by its objective. The straight chiropractic community had been doing it for some time now but it was the first time a national organization had undertaken to explain chiropractic by such a method. This removed many of the arbitrary aspects of chiropractic like "by hand only." While Reggie was influential and largely responsible for its formation and organization, and technically its only member from the time of incorporation until August, 1976, he chose to stay in the background, to not hold any office in the FSCO. Dr. Roger O'Dell of Michigan was elected the first president of the new organization.

That August day in Davenport, Iowa may have been the most significant day in the history of the straight chiropractic movement and the zenith of Reggie's public life. The straight chiropractic movement was truly born that day. It had been conceived during the past thirty-six months in Spartanburg, South Carolina in Reggie's mind. It had been nurtured in the hearts of hundreds of straight chiropractors, many of them members of the ICA and graduates of formerly straight schools. On that hot, humid afternoon as the meeting drew on, Thom Gelardi arrived and announced that the Board of Control, the governing body of the ICA had just voted to give $70,000 of the members' dues to the CCE to gain a seat on their board. There was nothing more to discuss or do, the FSCO was formed and the straight movement was officially born. While the organization has had its ups and downs and still is not a major force in the chiropractic community, its formation can be cited as the beginning of the straight chiropractic movement. Straight chiropractic had become more than a philosophy taught at a small college campus in South Carolina, it was now a political and organizational force. There was a place for all straight chiropractors, those that wanted chiropractic to be what B.J. envisioned and more, rather than less, to call home. Those straight chiropractors that had graduated from Palmer or National or Logan or Western States or New York or LACC now had a place to belong.

Immediately after the formation of the FSCO in Davenport, Iowa, Reggie sent out the following letter to chiropractors around the country:

> For many years now straight chiropractors have heeded the plaintive cry of "unity" and been lured into joining mixer organizations, hoping to change them. Thus they have not only given financial support to those who would sell our principle, but have disbanded their straight organizations, so that in many states there is no organization left to fight for good straight chiropractic legislation. The unified group in which the minority viewpoint is always outvoted, then presents to the legislative majority (mixer) viewpoint as being the only one, representing all of the chiropractors in the state. In short, the straight chiropractors have disenfranchised themselves.
>
> To make matters worse, the I.C.A., in order to attract membership has opened its doors to mixers, whose therapeutic practices are covered by I.C.A.'s vague "Chicago Definition," with the result that its policies now reflect the compromise viewpoint.
>
> The final and crushing blow came on August 20th, 1976 in the Sheraton Hotel in Rock Island, Illinois, where at its annual convention, I.C.A. Board of Control voted unanimously to pay $70,000 of your money (necessitating a dues increase) to the C.C.E. in exchange for one vote out of 15 on the C.C.E.
>
> The C.C.E. is an accrediting agency which, through heavy
>
> C.A. and other mixer political pressure has managed to have its stamp of approval recognized as a mandatory

prerequisite for any chiropractic college whose graduates wish to sit for licensure in most states. Masquerading as a legitimate accrediting agency, whose only interest is in upgrading the profession, C.C.E. has gained the support, or at least acquiescence, of even straight chiropractors. In fact, C.C.E. is the most powerful political tool of those who wish chiropractic to be absorbed into allopathic medicine. They are the number one enemy of the survival of straight chiropractic.

C.E. standards require that chiropractic colleges practice medical diagnosis in their clinics, and regard chiropractors as "diagnostic physicians whose primary purpose is to diagnose all patients for purposes of treatment and/or referral to other physicians."

Palmer College, Life College, and the Cleveland Colleges, thought by many to be among the last bastions of straight chiropractic, all now endorse C.C.E. and the therefore accept its doctrines, and now even the I.C.A. is putting its money (your money) and its support (your support) behind C.C.E.'s efforts to have chiropractic absorbed into medicine.

Sometimes coincidences of time are so fortuitous, that some see in them, divine intervention. Be that as it may, at the very moment that the I.C.A. in the Sheraton Hotel in Rock Island was making its decisions to join and support the enemy of our principle, across the river in Davenport, Iowaat the Clayton House Hotel a new group was forming dedicated to preserving that principle.

This new organization is the Federation of Straight Chiropractic Organizations. With straight groups organized in about twenty states already, they are a national and international voice for the pure principle of chiropractic.

This letter is to ask you to form a straight chiropractic association in your state, to get back your franchise and to show that there is an organized group that adheres to our true principles, and does not wish to go the path of the osteopath.

It is still not too late. Will you join us? Please answer today.

Yours for straight chiropractic,

Reginald R. Gold, D.C., Ph.C., F.I.C.A.
Executive Director

The "Hour Has Struck" is thought by some to be B.J. Palmer's high-water mark. That Lyceum in 1924, when he introduced the controversial NCM, may have been the zenith of his position in the straight chiropractic community. From that day on B.J.'s influence waned. It may be that the formation of the FSCO in 1976 was Reggie's high-water mark. He was articulate that day and he has been articulate many times since then. He has managed to rally people to a cause or to give great sums of money. Still today he has the ability to capture the undivided attention and admiration of the audience. But he did far more that day. It was not just a new organization or a new definition for chiropractic. It was a way of looking at chiropractic, from an objective standpoint that he developed not just for Sherman students and graduates but for all chiropractors. From that day on, the profession of chiropractic would never be the same. Whether the FSCO continued or continues as a force, whether Sherman stayed straight or not, a significant change had been made in the thinking of the profession. Chiropractors who reasoned deductively could never go back. Whether they will go forward and further expand the horizon of chiropractic remains to be seen. Reg made a contribution to chiropractic that day, a contribution of vision that has been dubbed "objective straight chiropractic," a vision on a par with D.D. adjusting Harvey Lillard and that perhaps has not been equaled since.

The years at Sherman were a good experience for Reggie even though unpleasant circumstances prompted his leaving. Interaction with students is always the most exciting aspect of a teaching experience. Students have an attitude about them that a philosopher loves. They ask questions simply for the sake of asking questions in the hope that they can win at the game of "stump the professor." Patients ask questions but nowhere near as often or as interesting as the ones the students ask. Basically, all patients ask the same 20 to 25 questions. Students, on the other hand, ask questions out of left field. So this was an especially important time for Reg and his development of the philosophy. It had to be able to stand up to critical scrutiny and students are an excellent source of that, especially when you are presenting something that is totally foreign to society, including the chiropractic community. Some of these students had come from traditional straight chiropractors' offices where the motto was "chiropractic gets sick people well." The chiropractor may have never heard Reggie's presentation or may not have yet grasped a total understanding of the non-therapeutic approach. Reg had only just begun to present this approach before going to Sherman and some had yet to get the idea. (Obviously, many in the profession still have not gotten it and continue to practice a semi-therapeutic approach to chiropractic).

It is also worthwhile to note that it was not only getting into teaching that was helpful to Reggie and his development of the philosophy but also getting out of practice. As philosophical as one might like to be in practice, patients often drag you down. You spend most of your time explaining chiropractic on the most basic level, so it is extremely difficult to expand your vision. It is like playing a sport with those of less skill, you cannot expect to improve, in fact the quality of your game may decrease. Well the same is true in practice. That may in part explain why so many chiropractors start off practicing philosophically and end up mixing. It is hard to stay focused while dealing with an outside-in thinking public every day. It is even more difficult to expand your vision. As great as Reggie's practical knowledge was, having built the largest chiropractic practice in the world, his real contribution occurred when he was able to step away from the day-to-day mundane aspects of practice and truly develop the philosophy. Sherman afforded him that opportunity and the straight chiropractic profession is fortunate for it. The profession is also fortunate that Reggie was willing to step into that thinking/teaching/apologist role. Many chiropractors who could make a contribution to the way the profession thinks and to the expansion of chiropractic philosophy, choose to stay in practice and make more money or put on practice-building seminars and make much more money. Reg did not and consequently made considerable financial sacrifices to broaden our understanding of chiropractic philosophy.

Despite the constant chaos of a new college and the crises that seemed to befall Sherman in those first few years, Reg had the opportunity to refine the philosophy both in the classroom and as he sat by his pool and contemplated the future of straight chiropractic. Reggie was fortunate in that he could make the transition from practitioner to instructor/administrator to political strategist in forming the FSCO. Part of that may have been natural ability or skills that he developed through his years in the military, but a large part of it was his focus on simplifying and communicating the chiropractic philosophy. He was always and is still trying to distill the chiropractic philosophy into its purest essence. That time was of tremendous importance to him, for the next two years were to be totally frustrating and thought consuming.

Despite his abrupt departure from Sherman, Reggie has nothing but fond remembrances of the school and Thom Gelardi. He feels that Sherman College has been without doubt the most important force in the development of straight chiropractic, at least the objective aspect of it. This accounts for his unswerving commitment to Sherman despite the school's compromises in recent years. Sherman was the place where Reg was free to develop and teach the greatest advancements in the chiropractic philosophy, the non-therapeutic approach. The school became a rallying point for the entire straight chiropractic community in those early years of the movement's development. The need for a school, the desire to keep it going and just the knowledge that there was an institution of higher learning that represented the objective straight approach was enough to keep many chiropractors involved with the movement who otherwise might have dropped out.

When Sherman began in 1972, the CCE was not yet recognized as an accrediting agency by the federal government. While Palmer and the Cleveland schools were not as straight as they should be, many saw hope for them to turn around and regain their former vision. When the CCE gained recognition that hope was all but lost. Sherman fought it rather than, like the other schools, teach diagnosis as the CCE said it should be taught. Sherman would and still teaches diagnosis so graduates can pass licensing exams. But unlike the traditional straight schools, Sherman has never tried to justify medical procedures as part of chiropractic. Reg felt that Sherman could be "Palmer as it should have been." It was the kind of school his alma mater would have been if all the changes that began after B.J.'s death had not occurred, changes that would have broken the Developer's heart. Sherman became a model for those other schools, a model of what they should be. Sherman continues to be that. There would be no doubt in the mind of anyone who would objectively watch the changes taking place in the chiropractic profession that^herman College has been a steadying force and has slowed the downward spiral of chiropractic. Sherman's approach to chiropractic has been a conscience to those who would compromise away everything that chiropractic has stood for since the days of the Palmers. So while the other schools attacked Sherman's unwillingness to give in as they had, they also admired the school for taking a stand. But Reg's thinking was that the profession or at least a great percentage of it would see the direction that Sherman had chosen to go and the direction the other schools were going and decide that Sherman represented the logical approach, in keeping with B.J.'s intent. Sherman would be a leader within the straight chiropractic profession. With this in mind it is understandable that he had a tremendous interest and concern for the school and an abiding love for it.

Among Reggie's fondest memories of Sherman is the College's first Lyceum. There had not been a chiropractic college Lyceum since the death of B.J. Dave Palmer immediately began to call the annual gathering "Homecoming." It was not the same. Beside B.J.'s absence, was missing the excitement, the fervor, the revival and the atmosphere complete with tent where chiropractors could rededicate themselves to the mission of taking chiropractic to the world. For a number of years, Reggie and others had tried to keep the Lyceum spirit alive at Palmer Homecoming. One year, the year the Anton Meister Auditorium, now the Alumni Auditorium, was completed, Reggie had given his now classic "Valley of the Blind" talk in the morning. Throughout the day word was spread around the school that Reggie would be doing a philosophy session at 9:00 pm. By that hour, the classroom that held 350 students and the adjoining one were filled to overflowing and people were still coming in. Irene called Dave Palmer and explained that their were almost 1500 people trying to get in the classroom and that they needed the new auditorium. Dave reluctantly agreed and so a procession of students, chiropractors, and other interested parties marched down the street to the large building. For the first hour, the sound system would not work, so Reggie had to practically scream to be heard in the large hall. He spoke for four hours. The feeling among the group was something very special. Most of these students were getting very little in the way of B.J. Philosophy. Irene's voice still rises with excitement as she relates that incident. Reggie recalls that event as one of the highlights of his life.

Sherman's first Lyceum recaptured some of that spirit. The students were as dedicated a group of people as could be found anywhere in the world. They were on a mission, sent to Sherman by dedicated straight chiropractors. They had no loans, no accreditation and at that point no assurance of getting a license anywhere when they graduated. The college had yet to erect permanent buildings for the school but they did have a piece of property. On Saturday night of that first Lyceum, on a clearing which would eventually be where the school stands today, a large bonfire was set and those students, faculty and chiropractors gathered to celebrate not the continuation of a chiropractic tradition but the rebirth of something, something that had literally died in the profession. After almost twenty-five years, Reg still gets emotional as he recalls the spirit, the love and the commitment that sparked the fire of that first Sherman Lyceum.

Reg's most joyful memory of Sherman is just in reflecting upon the growth of the college and knowing he contributed to that growth. Seeing those who were students at Sherman during his time there who now are leaders in the chiropractic profession and are keeping the torch of straight chiropractic lit is a fragrant memory. As teachers, mentors, and state association leaders they assure the passage of that torch on to future generations. One of Reg's characteristics is his ability to focus on those that are having a positive effect upon the chiropractic profession and not be discouraged about those that did not get the big idea. When he talks about his students, you would think that every one of them is out there helping to build straight chiropractic, although he acknowledges some monumental failures, Sherman grads who are out in practice as mixers. But even with those failures, he believes students who were there for the right reason are responsible for the caliber of Sherman graduates in practice today. Along those lines, Reggie is concerned about the type of student enrolling at Sherman now that it has accreditation. While there will be those who are dedicated and sent by dedicated chiropractors, there will be others who will come for reasons like location, conveniences, small classes and low cost of living.

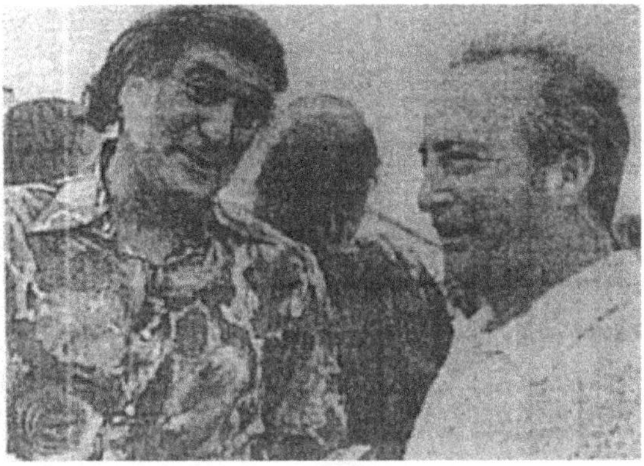

Reggie and the late Stephen Duff, D.C. enjoy a moment together at Lyceum

With the formation of the FSCO and his departure from Sherman, Reg Gold was ready for the next major phase of his life, despite the fact that he had yet to know what it was. He was developing audiovisual tools for chiropractors and he was constantly refining and simplifying the new objective straight chiropractic approach. He was doing seminars all over the world using ADIO House as his base of operations. He was also waiting for another ADIO to beckon him.

CHAPTER 4

ADIO Institute

1977-1979

By the middle of the 1970's it was common knowledge within the straight chiropractic community that a sister school to Sherman College would be started. The overall strategy was to have two or more straight colleges and then begin an accrediting agency that would perform all the functions that the CCE did for its member schools. At least one other school was absolutely necessary before the accrediting agency could be formed. The only questions were when and where it would begin and, of course, who would run it. Barbara Tompkins, who had been married to Dr. Carl Tompkins of Peekskill, New York approached Reggie at a Sherman Lyceum in 1976. Barbara, while not a chiropractor, was as strong a chiropractic advocate as any chiropractor could be. Reggie indicated that he would be willing to begin and run the school if she could organize a core group of supporters to help. Barbara was an avid chiropractic person and along with a few others began to look around the Northeastern part of the country. The tri-state area of New York, New Jersey and Pennsylvania was without doubt, the strongest straight chiropractic area in the country. This was in no small part due to the influence that Reggie had had during his years in Spring Valley. There were also a number of other important factors. Pennsylvania was a strong state for principled straight chiropractic. In the mid-sixties, when the state was battling the anti-advertising laws, the Chiropractic Fellowship of Pennsylvania, a new state organization began. Its leader was Dr. Clark Rich, a Palmer graduate from Clearfield, PA and one of the most successful and respected chiropractors in the state. Clark had one of the largest straight practices in the state. Although he was a regular attendee at D.E., he was respected by everyone in the straight chiropractic community. A soft spoken, unassuming person, Dr. Rich as President of the Chiropractic Fellowship of Pennsylvania, was the most influential straight chiropractor in Pennsylvania. Most of the organization's members were loyal to D.E., Sid Williams and the newly formed Life College. But they were also loyal to straight chiropractic. The Fellowship had two seminar meetings each year. At one Sid was usually the main speaker. At the other, Reggie was almost always the main speaker, so he had a fairly close relationship with the organization. At this point the lines were not so clearly drawn between the "traditional" straights and what would become known as the "objective" straights. As an organization, the Fellowship never fully embraced ADIO Institute but there is no doubt that their strength prepared the soil of that state for the planting of a second straight school. Probably the biggest contribution they made was in opening the state to Sherman graduates and keeping it open to them. There were not many states that accepted Sherman graduates and Pennsylvania was not only one of the first but one of the few that gave the school uninterrupted approval. Sherman alumni formed the moral strength, the recruiting force and also filled the majority of the faculty positions for the formation of ADIO.

Monroe Schneier, a chiropractor from the Plarrisburg area was the Fellowship's lobbyist in the mid-seventies. He would prove to be a valuable asset to ADIO over the years. Other well-known chiropractors like Jim Sigafoose and Wes Trout helped make the state of Pennsylvania very attractive for the opening of a new school. Reggie was usually a speaker on Wes' Living Principles Program and was a good friend of Dr. Trout's. Jim Sigafoose had also been greatly influenced by Reggie and had even adopted the "box on the wall" fee system that Reg had made famous. The north and central

New Jersey areas were probably filled with the strongest group of straight chiropractors in the country, many of whom had been part of the Saturday night groups in Spring Valley. New Jersey chiropractors like Jim Doherty, Joe Donofrio, Ron Peak, Marty Brown, Tony Demarco and Lou Pannucio made the eastern part of Pennsylvania the more likely place to start the school, so that their strength and support could be utilized. Finally, in May of 1977, a group of chiropractors and other interested parties approached Reggie at another Sherman Lyceum and asked him to come to the Philadelphia area and start a school. This group included Tedd Koren, David Blessing, a lay person, Carl Savio, and a few others. Everyone knew it was Reggie who was the most likely person to begin the school and they wanted him to stay on as President. He had teaching experience at Columbia and Sherman and administrative experience at Sherman. Other than traveling around to do weekend seminars, he had no commitments that would tie him down. Besides, Reg was the most recognizable figure in the straight chiropractic community and his association with any school would guarantee that hundreds of chiropractors would refer students there. The idea of learning philosophy from Reggie Gold was a major reason why hundreds of students had been referred to Sherman, a brand new school with no accreditation and only a few states open to its graduates. Most of Sherman's students had come from and were still coming from the New York, New Jersey and Pennsylvania area despite the fact that New York and New Jersey were not open to Sherman graduates at the time (although, many felt that it was only a matter of time until New Jersey was open). Pennsylvania was already open so prospective students from three states saw ADIO as an opportunity to attend a straight school without having to move to South Carolina for three years, something that was not particularly attractive to many northerners. Reggie and the founders of ADIO were sure that the Pennsylvania school could attract even more students than Sherman.

In July of 1977, Reggie moved into the Philadelphia area to begin the school. He rented a very modest home in the Junewood section of Levittown about a mile from where the school would open.

Irene was by this time an important member of the faculty and administration at Sherman. Since there was not really a teaching position for Irene at ADIO with only one matriculated class, she stayed in South Carolina. Reggie met with a group of interested chiropractors in the lecture room of my chiropractic office in Levittown, Pennsylvania in July. The group included some former students of Reggie's at Columbia, like Joe Donofrio and myself, students from Sherman, like Tedd Koren and Claude Lessard, and a number of other interested chiropractors. During that first meeting Reggie suggested the name "ADIO College of Straight Chiropractic" and everyone enthusiastically agreed. Soon after, however, it was learned that a school could not call itself a college unless it was approved by the Pennsylvania Department of Education (D.O.E.), something that would take the school almost six years to accomplish, long after Reggie's departure. The obstacle to acquiring college status from the D.O.E. was the obtainment of a $500,000 endowment. This was a fund that the D.O.E. required for all colleges. It had to be unencumbered, although the school could use the interest earned on it. Reggie and the others at that meeting decided that a major fund-raising campaign would be undertaken to raise $800,000. $300,000 would go toward getting the school off the ground, a figure Reg felt was reasonable, and the remaining

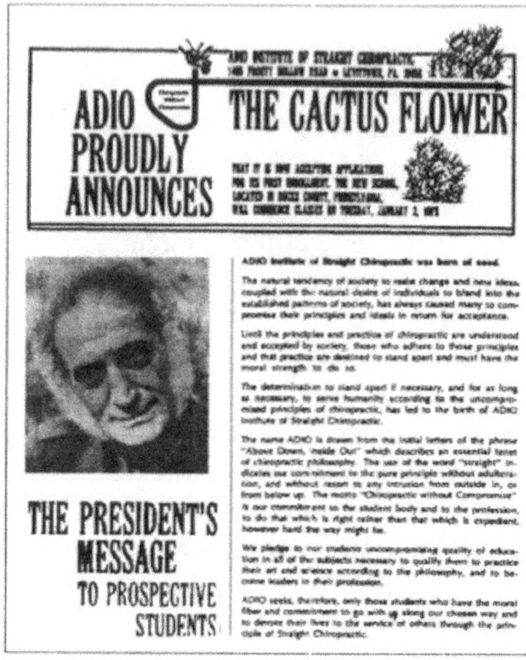

ADIO PROUDLY ANNOUNCES

THE CACTUS FLOWER

THE PRESIDENT'S MESSAGE TO PROSPECTIVE STUDENTS

ADIO Institute of Straight Chiropractic was born of need.

The natural tendency of society to resist change and new ideas, coupled with the natural desire of individuals to blend into the established patterns of society, has always caused many to compromise their principles and ideals in return for acceptance.

Until the principles and practice of chiropractic are understood and accepted by society, those who adhere to those principles and that practice are destined to stand apart and must have the moral strength to do so.

The determination to stand apart if necessary, and for as long as necessary, to serve humanity according to the uncompromised principles of chiropractic, has led to the birth of ADIO Institute of Straight Chiropractic.

The name ADIO is drawn from the initial letters of the phrase "Above Down, Inside Out" which describes an essential tenet of chiropractic philosophy. The use of the word "straight" indicates our commitment to the pure principle without adulteration, and without resort to any intrusion from outside in, or from below up. The motto "Chiropractic without Compromise" is our commitment to the student body and to the profession, to do that which is right rather than that which is expedient, however hard the way might be.

We pledge to our students uncompromising quality of education in all of the subjects necessary to qualify them to practice their art and science according to the philosophy, and to become leaders in their profession.

ADIO seeks, therefore, only those students who have the moral fiber and commitment to go with us along our chosen way and to devote their lives to the service of others through the principle of Straight Chiropractic.

ADIO Institute of Straight Chiropractic announces its opening in its publication, The Cactus Flower

$500,000. would be placed into the endowment fund. To raise this figure, it was suggested that 100 chiropractors would be solicited to each give $8,000. They would be designated forever as Founders of the College. Apparently, Reggie and the rest of the schools' organizers did not see this figure as a formidable barrier to the development of the school. With all the straight chiropractors around the country, all the people that knew and respected Reggie and the knowledge that a second school was needed, everyone felt that the figure could be reached. Unfortunately, it was not to be. Reggie had been a great fund-raiser for Sherman. However, the day-to-day activities that were required to get the school opened prevented him from traveling around the country to raise funds for ADIO. A number of other factors significantly effected the fund-raising efforts for ADIO. For example, many of the ADIO supporters were young Sherman graduates who were just struggling to get their practices off the ground and could not afford to give $80, let alone $8,000. Other chiropractors had a "wait and see" attitude about the school, knowing all the problems Sherman was having in getting its graduates licensed in more than a handful of states. Many who did regularly contribute to the straight chiropractic profession, wanted to make sure it went to a viable institution and so they continued to give to Sherman only.

Despite the slowly growing list of Founders (the school would close in 1995 without ever reaching its goal of 100), Reggie and the others pushed to open the school. The faculty and administration was largely composed of young, inexperienced chiropractors and it was up to Reggie to keep them focused, enthused and committed to the task of building a straight chiropractic educational institution and its importance to the future of straight chiropractic. The straight chiropractic leadership decided that it would begin to develop an accrediting agency to provide an alternative to the CCE. Already, Reggie and others were preparing to form just such an agency as soon as the second school, ADIO, was functioning. Most of the first faculty consisted of recent Sherman graduates. Tedd Koren, who had a year or two earlier begun a practice in the Philadelphia area, was asked to join the staff. Ben Tanner, a graduate of the pioneer class at Sher-

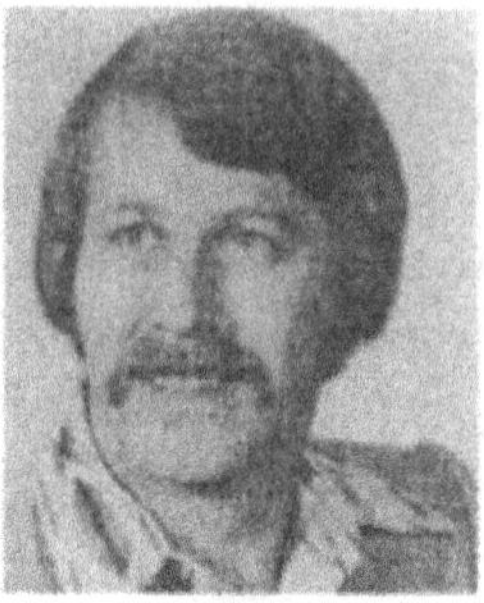

Dr. Joe Strauss
Spinal Anatomy

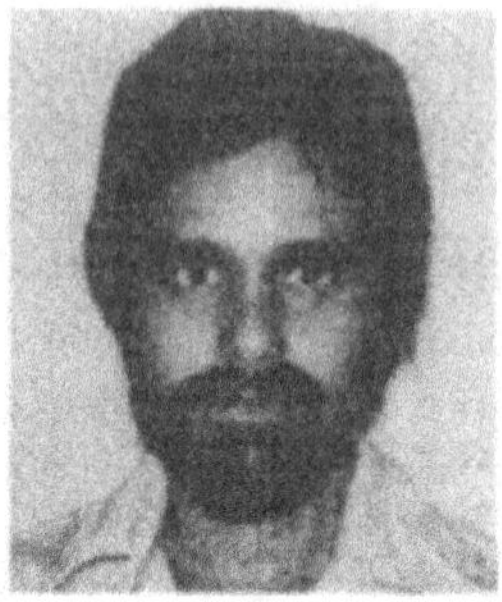

Dr. Ted Koren
Histology and Technic

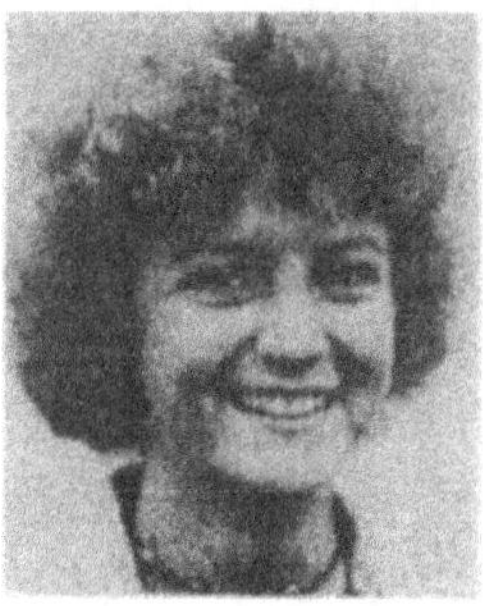

Dr. P.J. Martin
Osteology and Technic

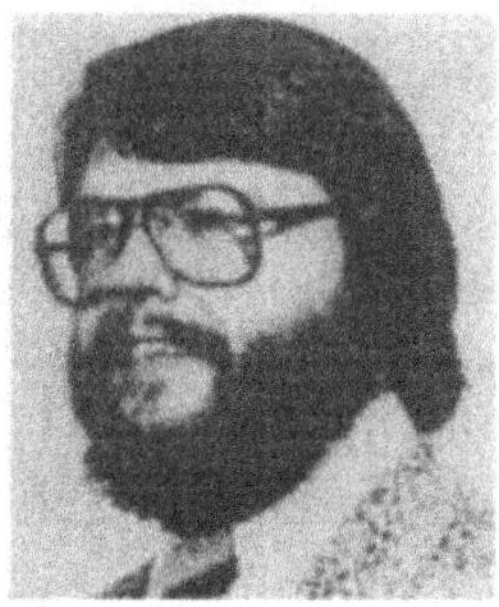

Dr. Claude Lessard
Technic

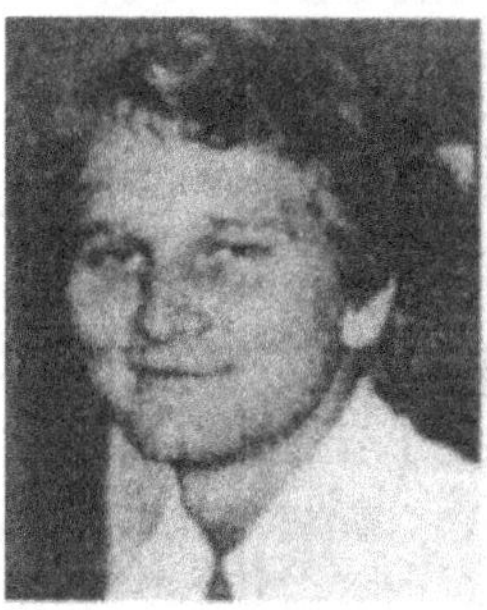

Dr. Ben Tanner
Technic

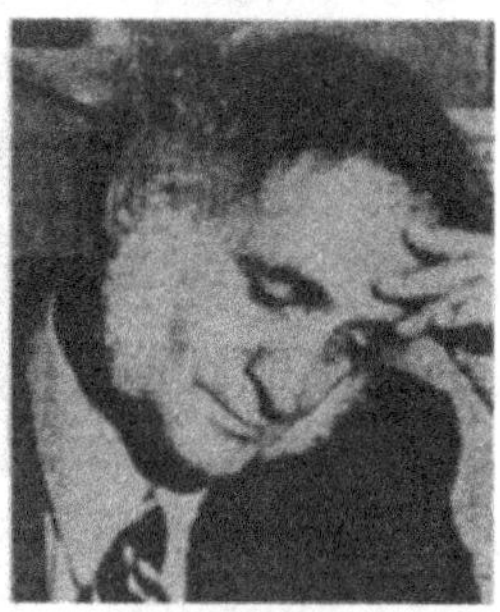

Dr. Reg Gold
Philosophy and Terminology

The first faculty members of ADIO Institute

man and originally from Bucks County just north of Philadelphia, was asked to teach technique. He had been practicing in nearby Newtown, PA since his graduation from Sherman in 1976. P.J. Martin, who had been living in the Spartanburg area moved up to the Philadelphia area to teach and begin a practice. P.J. was one of Reggie's most ardent supporters and wanted to help Reggie in getting the new school started. Claude Lessard, a recent Sherman graduate originally from Canada, had already moved to the area anticipating the opening of the school. Both Martin and Lessard were asked to teach technique. Reggie, of course, taught Philosophy and I, the only non-Sherman graduate besides Reggie, taught Spinal Anatomy. Reggie's concept of a chiropractic faculty was somewhat different than the rest of the world's and it would later prove to be a major conflict at ADIO and in fact, prompt his departure. Reggie believed that faculty members should be successful practitioners (or at least moving towards success) and that they should donate their teaching time. He felt that full-time faculty did not have the practice experience that benefited the students and that those that did not practice could easily lose their vision, without the day-to-day contact with real patients. Paying a faculty would discourage them from practicing. (Author's Note: Having taught at a chiropractic college and also built and sustained a large practice, quite frankly, it is easier to teach than to build and sustain a practice. The chiropractor who teaches has guaranteed salary, usually health benefits and paid holidays. It can be a comfortable life.) However, it can also lead to a lack of motivation and that was what Reg didn't want.

There was no doubt that Reg's faculty was motivated, energetic and enthusiastic. Unfortunately, other than myself, none of them had built practices. During a meeting, just before the opening of the school, I approached the subject of salary with Reg because a number of the faculty had asked me about it. Reg had been their teacher, actually a teacher to all of us, although myself some thirteen years before the others and they were reluctant to ask about money, not wanting Reg to think they were in it for financial gain, which they were not. Reg made it clear that he had no intention of paying the faculty. No one said a word and the meeting continued. Later, a number of the chiropractors indicated to me that they were surprised that they were not going to be paid but that teaching under Reggie was enough payment and they took the job anyhow.

Despite opposition to the development of the school, plans progressed. When Sherman opened in 1973, the mixing/straight battle was not much more than a dislike for one another and the straight chiropractic community was fairly united. That is, those that supported Sid Williams and his approach also supported the opening of Sherman. That was the early seventies. It was not so much that Sherman sneaked in before the mixers realized it, but that the mixers were largely impotent when Sherman began. After the inception of Sherman, the CCE, which for many years had been the ACA's accrediting agency, received recognition from the federal government.

This not only gave the mixers tremendous power but it also rendered the straight schools powerless and forced them to capitulate. Sherman began on neutral ground. ADIO began after the camps had already divided. Sherman was on their side, but everybody else was on the side of the CCE either by desire or coercion. By 1977, the war had heated up. The leadership in the mixing community knew where the straights were coming from or more appropriately, where they were going. It was understood that the straight movement saw chiropractic for everyone, not just those with disease conditions. Further, the mixers understood that the ultimate goal was to flood the country with straight chiropractors. This would create economic problems for the mixer inasmuch as it would increase competition. What was even worse, it could upset the political balance, creating a potential force of straights who might one day influence legislation to outlaw mixing. Beside the political factor, there was also the "patient safety" factor. Most of the mixing community still viewed the "Sherman straights" and the "Life straights" as the same. While most of them did not care for Sid Williams and his brand of philosophy, he at least did not oppose the CCE and its emphasis on diagnosis. So the mixers viewed Reggie, Thom and their followers as chiropractors who thought they could cure everything, in every person (the Life College philosophy) without doing any screening procedures (diagnosis). If Sid was radical, then Reggie's group was radical and dangerous.

The five years subsequent to the formation of Sherman had helped to define and solidify the straight chiropractic that Reggie was presenting to the profession. It was not dangerous because the patient was informed that the treatment of medical problems was not the objective of the straight chiropractor and that the diagnosis or treatment of a condition, if desired, should be sought from another health care provider. Whether this approach to chiropractic was ever understood by the general mixing community is open to discussion. By this time the lines had been clearly drawn. CCE had been recognized. Sherman had applied to it, been turned down, sued the CCE and indicated that they were withdrawing their application and would not re-apply because the CCE did not have the same chiropractic objectives as they did. (The objective of straight chiropractic is to correct vertebral subluxation regardless of the medical condition, not to treat it, but to allow the body to work closer to its potential.) Of course, that objective was unacceptable to the CCE, at least at that time. The diagnosis issue has since become very clearly defined, largely due to Reg's persistent articulation of the subject and his ability to bring out the simple logic of his position. Diagnosis was shown to be inconsistent with the chiropractic objective and the use of it not only illogical but counterproductive to everything that the straight chiropractor was trying to accomplish. This was the issue that began to bitterly divide the straight chiropractic community which had formerly been united by their position against modalities. Between the beginning of Sherman and that of ADIO, Life College had been formed with perhaps more support both financially and in the referring of students than any other school in chiropractic history. Life and its founder Sid Williams had decided very early to be a CCE school, to incorporate medical diagnosis in the curriculum and to justify its being done in a chiropractic office. During this time Sid had also carried out his plan to gain control of the ICA. Other than a failed attempt by some members to merge the organization with the ACA, Sid's takeover went smoothly.

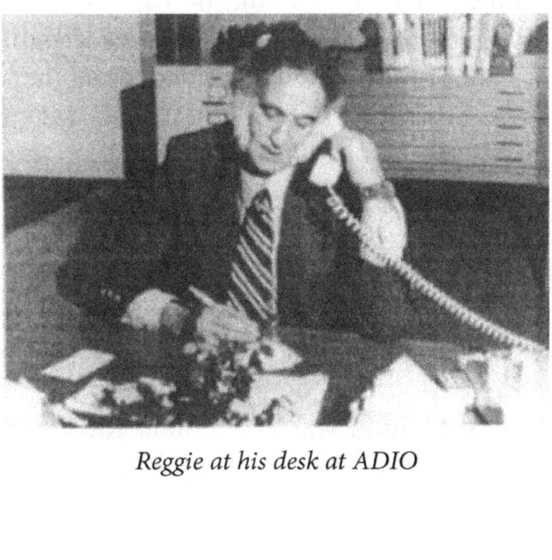

Reggie at his desk at ADIO

With all of the above factors and events, the environment in which ADIO began was quite different than that in which Sherman had started five years earlier. With the opening of ADIO, the financial drain on the straight chiropractic community doubled as its numbers dwindled due to the schism caused by the diagnosis issue. The straight chiropractic community was clearly divided between Sid and the traditional straights who became known as Palmer/Life/ICA straights and Reggie and Thom and the Sherman/ADIO/FSCO straights. Some chiropractors threw their support to Sid, many of the straights, sick over the internecine straight battles, stopped supporting either. Many straights were also being lured from straight chiropractic altogether by the insurance dollars that modalities were bringing during that period. And, of course, Sherman College had not yet been in existence long enough to begin to resupply the straight chiropractic community with chiropractors who were able to financially help the cause. All of this made it a very hostile environment in which Reggie and the founders of ADIO began to work.

Despite all the obstacles, the school opened it doors in January 1978, less than six months after Reggie had been asked to head it up. That alone bespeaks the energy and the persistence of the man. He began with virtually no funds, a very modest salary and the help of just a few practicing chiropractors who helped to locate a building for classrooms and to spread the word. For almost a year from the time of its conception, Reggie was the only full-time and only paid administrator of the school. On the first day of the school's opening, a small ceremony took place in one of the school's classrooms, which was a small wing of an elementary school, the Ralph Waldo Emerson School in Levittown. Bristol Township students were still attending classes in the remainder of the school. At the opening ceremony, Thom Gelardi spoke as did the chairman of the Board of Trustees from Sherman, Earl Taylor, who sadly passed away a few days later. After the ceremony, a luncheon meeting was held at a nearby restaurant. At that time, Reggie was formally installed as president of ADIO Institute of Straight Chiropractic. Prior to that, Joe Donofrio had been elected Chairman of the Board of Trustees of ADIO and I had been elected Vice-Chairman.

The Pioneer Class had twenty-four students. Some of them were there because the school's location was convenient for them, but all of them were there to be taught philosophy by Reggie. Reg was under a tremendous handicap trying to teach, do administrative work and raise funds all at the same time. Despite the fact that teaching five days a week kept Reggie from traveling to promote the school and that money was slow coming in, the school continued and grew. It is a tremendous credit to Reg Gold that twenty-four students began the ADIO program in January and that about fifty more started in the next eight months. There were no other well-known chiropractors associated with the school at the time. It was not accredited. Not only was it not accredited, it had been made clear from the outset that it had no intention of applying to the CCE. The incorporation of SCASA was still six months away when the school opened, although Reg began working on the charter and by-laws as soon as ADIO opened. The CCE, the mixers and even the ICA straights were attempting to tie the noose tighter and tighter around the neck of Sherman. Graduates had gotten into the state of Pennsylvania based upon the school's approval by the now defunct accrediting agency of the ICA. This agency had at one time been in competition with the CCE for federal recognition, but when the Federal Government recognized the CCE, all the ICA schools (e.g., Palmer, Cleveland, Logan) applied to it and the ICA's accrediting agency just withered away. Fortunately for Sherman, the state of Pennsylvania had approved Sherman graduates for licenses while this accrediting agency was still in existence. The mixers were putting pressure on the state of Pennsylvania to rescind Sherman's approval. But either way, ADIO could not get its graduates approved for licensing on that basis. To further complicate matters, since there had been no new schools in over twenty-five years, the state of Pennsylvania had no mechanism to approve a school. Inasmuch as CCE was now in place, there was no need to have a procedure for approving chiropractic colleges except for ADIO. New schools from this point on would be approved or not based upon CCE guidelines. But ADIO was there and would not be ignored, although that is exactly what the Pennsylvania State Board attempted to do. In February, as chief executive officer, Reggie wrote the state board explaining that a new school had started (as if they did not know) and inquired what it would take to achieve approval by the Board. It was fortunate for ADIO that the bureaucracy of state governments moves so slowly. The State board still had provisions to individually approve chiropractic colleges although accreditation by the CCE was the mechanism by which all the other colleges had gained approval in Pennsylvania, except for Sherman. To be approved directly by the state board was the hope that Reggie and the student body held onto pending the recognition by the federal government of a straight accrediting agency equivalent to the CCE.

The slowness of state bureaucracy, however, was a double-edged sword. While it had left the door open for ADIO's approval, it also made the process of getting state approval slower than death. Whether it was purposeful on the part of the mixers on the board, mere government incompetence or ignorance as to what to do with the first chiropractic college in the state in modem times is open to conjecture. Reg made an application to the state board in February of 1978, one month after the school opened. Since there was no formal application process, the application consisted of a letter listing the school's faculty and objectives and asking for information and guidelines for approval. It was not until the fall of 1979 that the State board sent guidelines and then only after the threat of legal action.

Lack of leadership has always been one of the great problems in the chiropractic profession. During the developmental period of the objective straight chiropractic philosophy, 1972-1987, this lack of leadership was very obvious. In the mid-seventies, the decision making was almost entirely done by Reggie and Thom. Occasionally others were called for help or input, people like Joe Donofrio and Leonard Rutherford. The overall plan was to have two or more schools, and then a separate accrediting agency to rival the CCE. Beyond that there was no real long range planning. In the back of everyone's mind was the hope that one day there could be two professions, one to serve straight chiropractic and the other to serve those who wanted to take chiropractic more and more into medicine. So there were some long-range goals, but the day to day carrying out of projects and activities to achieve this long-range goal was just that, day-to-day decisions. Everyone in the movement was flying by the seat of their pants. The philosophy was still evolving and the communication of it to the field was a slow process. Reggie could not be everywhere putting on seminars to bring people along to where he was taking the philosophy and, of course, there was a tremendous amount of resistance to change by many straights. Some had a difficult time moving away from the ideas of their alma mater, the Founder, their friends and/or their state or national association. It was a period of prosperity for most straight chiropractors, actually for most chiropractors in general, and it was difficult for them to see that there was no future in their approach. They could not grasp the fact that addressing medical conditions with chiropractic to get insurance dollars held no future in the long run.

In 1978, Reggie organized the World Congress on the Future of Straight Chiropractic in Washington, D.C. Reggie met with Thom Gelardi and others in the nation's capital to discuss matters pertinent to the two schools and the straight movement. The significance of the Congress was the document produced by it called, "Excerpts From the Proceedings of the 1978 World Congress on the Future of Straight Chiropractic." The original purpose of the document was to have something to present to the federal government to demonstrate the straight chiropractic viewpoint and how it differed from the CCE model. The 42-page document, presented in a booklet form, is significant because it represented the first, and what would be for the next thirteen years, the only formal document addressing the practice of objective straight chiropractic. The first of the four essays is entitled "Consumer Rights in Chiropractic" and it bears the authorship of Reginald R. Gold, D.C., Ph.C., F.I.C.A. The first section deals with safety with respect to technique, case history, physical examination, spinographic x-ray study and consultation and judgment. Having read this section of the document for the first time in almost eighteen years, I was struck by how clearly and succinctly it explains the chiropractic philosophy as it pertains to case management today. I am not sure I myself really grasped the breadth nor the accuracy with which this document presented the objective straight chiropractic position when it was first published.

Reg makes important points in each of the above areas, but perhaps the essence of the approach that Reg and the straight movement had developed is found under the heading of Physical Examination. He specifies that the examination is done to analyze the spine to determine "whether an adjustment is needed, and if so, where and how." Second, the physical examination is done to determine whether "any technique of choice may be contra-indicated by the presence of physical factors." Notice Reg does not say whether chiropractic is needed, it is assumed if the first criteria is met (i.e., if a subluxation is present) that chiropractic care is indicated. The determination is whether there is a contradiction to a certain technique. Just to make sure that the reader and the entire profession is aware of the objective straight approach, Reggie adds the following, "N.B. AT NO TIME SHOULD A CHIROPRACTOR HOLD HIMSELF OR HERSELF OUT TO BE COMPETENT TO DETERMINE WHETHER OR NOT ANY PATIENT MAY BE IN NEED OF ANY THERAPEUTIC SERVICES." In the next two paragraphs he expands upon the statement, "Whether or not a disease is present, and whether or not a therapy may be desirable to treat any such disease, is irrelevant to the practice of chiropractic." He goes on to explain that every person experiences life better without subluxations and that for a chiropractor to claim to be as competent as a physician "in the diagnosis and treatment of disease... constitutes the most blatant form of quackery and consumer fraud." Under the section, "Freedom of Choice and The Consumer's Right to Know," Reggie explains that straight chiropractic does not relate to the treatment, cure or prevention of disease in any way and that it is the chiropractor's responsibility to make the patient aware of his or her unique objective.

The fact that this document has been made public since 1978 makes a strong statement about the mixing aspect of the profession. Time and again they decry our approach saying we want to take care of every disease or that we believe subluxation is the cause of all disease. Those who have in this way misrepresented the objective straight chiropractic position from the platform, in print or before legislative and governmental bodies, can only have done so for one of two reasons. Either they never read this document, in which case they were remiss in commenting on an approach of which they were totally ignorant by choice, or they understood our unique approach and purposely distorted it. Anyone who presents a viewpoint especially in rebutting it, has a obligation to have a reasonable amount of knowledge on the subject. From 1978 until at least 1991, this was the definitive explanation of the objective straight approach. One can only conclude that those who comment on objective straight chiropractic and distort its purpose are either academically and intellectually incompetent or they are ethically bankrupt. The position is there, it is clear for anyone to read and I, for one, can find no other possible explanation for the preposterous charges that have been leveled against straight chiropractors, their schools and their accrediting agency over the last eighteen plus years.

The remainder of the excerpts while under the byline of other people unmistakably manifest Reggie's influence. "The Role of Chiropractic in Tomorrow's Health" contrasts the ADIO viewpoint of health and the outside-in viewpoint. "The Goals of Chiropractic Education" is intended to demonstrate to legislative, accrediting and governmental agencies the logic and the competency of a straight chiropractic education.

The last article is titled, "The Future of Straight Chiropractic." This essay presents the different scenarios of chiropractic should the mixing aspect of the profession prevail, the straights prevail or the profession continue in its present state. The fourth alternative, the one that Reggie and the rest of the objective straight chiropractors would like to see, is a complete separation into two professions. That alternative has virtually been set aside in the last three years, despite the fact that it was the preferable option of the straight community in 1978.

During the early part of 1978, in addition to his duties at the school and doing seminars and chiropractic conventions on the weekends, as much as his schedule would allow, Reg began working on the development of the Straight Chiropractic Academic Standards Association (SCASA). This accrediting agency would reflect the objective straight approach to chiropractic that Reg and others had been developing since the early seventies. Now that ADIO was opened, it was time to begin the accreditation process. In June of 1978, six months after the opening of ADIO, Reg had lawyers in Harrisburg incorporate SCASA in the state of Pennsylvania. Of course, the incorporation was only the beginning. Bylaws needed to be drawn up and then the long arduous task of developing standards had to take place. These standards would be the guidelines for straight schools to follow and by which they would be evaluated. After the standards were developed, they had to be evaluated by a cross section of the straight chiropractic community, both educators and practicing chiropractors. Then changes and more changes would be made and finally, the schools would be apprised of the standards and given the opportunity to apply for accreditation. Meanwhile, the Department of Education of the federal government was to be petitioned to recognize SCASA as an accrediting agency for straight chiropractic colleges.

The purpose of accreditation included allowing students to qualify for student loans. However, the fact that many states were allowing students to sit for the state board's examinations based upon their schools' accreditation made accreditation a much more important issue. The mixing aspect of the profession saw accreditation as the Achilles' heel of the straight chiropractic community. Consequently, they pressed the individual states to restrict licenses to only those schools that were accredited by an accrediting agency recognized by the federal government. As a result, each year the number of states open to Sherman graduates dwindled and, of course, the potential pool of new students shrank along with it. The outlook was even more bleak for potential ADIO graduates. "Grandfather laws" and the old ICA accreditation helped Sherman but not ADIO. When the first class of ADIO graduated in December of 1980, there were actually only two states open to them, Georgia and Michigan, and Georgia subsequently closed. An accrediting agency for the straight schools was an absolute necessity.

SCASA, although incorporated in June of 1978 did not become a viable accrediting agency for a number of years. It would be twelve years before it would finally gain recognition by the United States Department of Education and even that would be short-lived. In December of 1995, the Board of SCASA would vote to dissolve the accrediting agency apparently ending forever the dream of a separate vehicle for straight schools to gain federal government recognition.

Once Reg had gotten the accreditation ball rolling, he did not get involved in the process. It was turned over to professionals (or at least those that the straight community believed to be professionals) to organize and develop. His lack of involvement did not mean that he was relaxing. On the contrary, ADIO was becoming much more time consuming. To the 24 students in the January 1978 pioneer class were added a half dozen in the spring quarter, about 15 in the summer and well over 30 in the fall. It was truly amazing to see the numbers of students enrolling at ADIO in the first eighteen months. The school had no recognition, no accreditation and no assurance of licenses for its graduates anywhere except that Sherman graduates having the same practice objective, were getting into a few states. ADIO's second physical plant was another elementary school built in the 50's to absorb the baby boom and the migration to the suburbs which by the late seventies had waned. The school district was happy to rent the empty building out to ADIO. The school really had very little to offer students except for Reggie Gold. But that in and of itself was enough to attract scores of young people.

Reg traveled around the country doing other things for the straight chiropractic movement. He testified at the hearings in 1978 to review CCE's Commission of Accreditation recognition by the Federal Government. He testified on behalf of the FSCO, although at the time he was president of ADIO. During his testimony he made some interesting comments, the most intriguing of which was in the beginning. He said, "The chiropractic profession in recent years has divided itself very clearly into two camps, that which has become known as straight chiropractic and that which has been given to be called mixing. Now we take serious objection to the term mixing because it implies that the mixer mixes something with chiropractic." Reg is saying, perhaps so subtly that the government officials never picked up on it, that you cannot practice two diverse objectives and call it one profession, especially when there is already a licensed profession (medicine) practicing one of those objectives. That is exactly what the mixers were trying and continue to try to do. ADIO reflected Reggie's desires and objectives for a straight chiropractic education.

While Sherman College was still heavily emphasizing the upper cervical technique, ADIO was determined to also promote full-spine adjusting with the same fervor and specificity of the HIO technique. Reg saw the idea of a full-spine school as a challenge, friendly competition with Sherman and Thom. He also felt that despite the effectiveness of the HIO approach, the majority of the profession leaned toward full-spine adjusting and would prefer to send their students to a full-spine school. Even though Reg was in the first class at Palmer to be taught full-spine adjusting, it was not taught with much enthusiasm and upper cervical was still considered to be the only "straight" chiropractic technique. Interestingly, Reg later found that many of his upper cervical teachers actually practiced full spine in their private practices. He was trained in HIO work, but Reg graduated not being satisfied with upper cervical work for a living. Partially because he was dissatisfied with the logic of it. He recalls the day he asked B.J. why a subluxation can not occur below axis.

A. J.'s answer was, "because I said so." As much as Reg revered this man, the answer did not make sense. Without a logical explanation, Reg could not be satisfied that HIO was the way to go.

Not only was he not satisfied with the adjusting of only one or two segments, but the form of analysis that the upper cervical practitioners used did not make sense to him. Gonstead's full-spine analysis was not any more logical to him. The Mt. Horeb chiropractor said the subluxation was manifested by a hot spot due to capillary congestion at the site of the subluxation. As much as Reg respected Gonstead, that explanation left much to be desired. Reg knew that a subluxation could cause effects anywhere else so he did not accept

Gonstead's theory. Pierce later said it was due to capillary infarction, that the upper cervical region was actually a cold spot. B.J. said the purpose of the bipolar thermometer was to compare one side with the other, to see if there is consistency (a pattern) which would indicate that the body was not changing. Sameness in the graph reading indicates a lack of change, that the body is not adapting fully. Unfortunately, the instrument did not tell where the subluxation was. Other forms of analysis such as nerve tracing and the Meric System were symptom oriented and not helpful to someone who was looking for subluxation regardless of the absence or presence of symptoms. All of the systems that Reg investigated had their shortcomings, even the pattern work presented two great problems. Suppose a subluxation had been present for thirty or forty years and permanently damaged the nerve so that even though the subluxation was corrected, the nerve could never again carry the mental impulse and therefore give a false positive. Conversely, the body adapts in spite of the subluxation, just not as well, so a person could not be in pattern but still carrying nerve interference. The pattern is an effect that could indicate a subluxation anywhere. It is not a message from the body telling you where a subluxation is or if it is present at all.

When Reg began practicing he immediately began to work on his analysis. He knew that just structurally lining up bone, which was the first palpation used in chiropractic, was not effective because a straight spine is not necessarily free of subluxations, just as deviations from the average do not necessarily mean that the spine is subluxated. He began feeling bumps and muscles. He knew there were changes in the muscles but taut and tender fibers were possibly an effect rather than the body's attempt to correct a subluxation and hence something that could be analyzed. He knew that x-ray was only effective as an analytic tool on the first visit and could not be used on a regular basis. Besides, he was looking to get away from x-ray inasmuch as it was associated with medicine and was an invasive procedure. Many chiropractors were using a muscle palpation methodology which Reg eventually came to call "vertebraille." It is just an art form that evolved among chiropractors, many of whom probably do not even realize what they are doing or feeling. As Reg continued in practice, this system evolved and developed both as an art and as a systematic method. When Reg went to Sherman he began to formally systematize this subluxation analysis. At first it was done off campus with students who were interested in learning it at his home. Eventually he was permitted to bring it into the Sherman curriculum. Two students from Spain, Michelle and Miguel Bolufer, had a great interest in it. Miguel took extensive notes in class and put them together in a manual for other students. This was the first systematization of what became known as " muscle palpation."

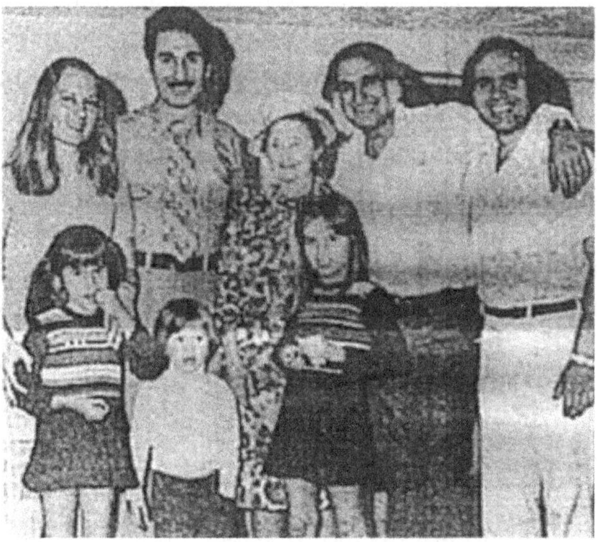

Michele and Miguel Bolufer and family pose with Reggie and Thom. They would return to Spain as chiropractors and eventually run the Spinal Tutorium for Reg.

The beauty of this system is that it is based on a philosophical, deductive concept. The reasoning, reduced to as simple an explanation as possible, is that the body "hates" vertebral subluxations and the innate intelligence will make every effort to reduce them as quickly as possible. Further, it is deduced that since the musculature system is the major system used by the body to correct them, one should be able to develop the palpatory skills to tell which muscles are trying to move which bones and in what specific direction. A knowledge of muscle anatomy, the origin and insertion of the muscles, would obviously be a necessary component to locate subluxations by this method. The principle is that the muscle would be "working" to correct the subluxation, but because of the nerve interference in that "vertemere" it does not have sufficient energy to do it. The chiropractor assesses where more force is needed and introduces minimal force with the proper line of drive to allow the body's innate intelligence to take the force and correct the vertebral subluxation. It is a rather simple idea, yet brilliant. It may not have even been a new idea. Many chiropractors were using it to some degree or another although they did not realize what they were doing. Reg began to categorize and define the system or at least set people in the direction of being able to develop it. Nick Spano, D.C. has probably done the most work in documenting and teaching the system in his seminars. Nick was a student at ADIO and learned the basics of the muscle palpation system there. Later, as Reg developed Spinology, the system would be extremely important because the Spinologist would have no other tools (e.g., x-ray or NCM) at his or her disposal. Many people are completely unaware that Reggie is responsible for this significant contribution to the art of chiropractic. Muscle palpation is a fine system of analysis, unfortunately, learning the art of it is time consuming. It takes years of practice to sensitize the fingers to know what you are feeling. And of course it is a very subjective form of analysis.

While ADIO was a full-spine school, that did not mean that upper-cervical work was set aside. On the contrary, Reggie was determined that the graduates of ADIO would be able to hold their own in the analysis and adjustment of the Atlas/Axis with any student from Sherman. P.J. Martin taught upper cervical adjusting to the first quarter students. As a Sherman graduate, she was proficient in the technique and determined that her students would be also. Of all the faculty, P.J. probably recognized better than anyone what Reg was trying to accomplish with the school. Her loyalty to Reggie was unswerving. She was a loyal faculty member till the day he left the school, then she too resigned and followed him into Spinology. Eventually she ran the San Francisco Tutorium until it closed. At the time of this writing, she is back in chiropractic college to get the credits necessary to practice in California where she resides with her husband, who is also a children. California would not recognize her degree from Sherman College. P.J. had an ear-piercing clap. She used it to drill the first quarter students in their toggle. While it was assumed that very few of the ADIO graduates would practice HIO and that most would probably never toggle in practice, the technique developed coordination, speed, muscle control and discipline. Those qualities are desirable no matter what technique a chiropractor uses and Reg felt toggle recoil adjusting helped develop them.

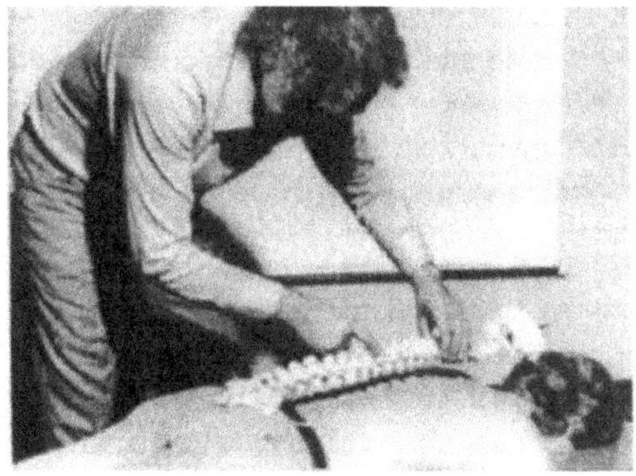

Reggie explaining a technique concept to an early chiropractor, and their class at ADIO

With regard to x-ray analysis, Reggie wanted to not only equal Sherman but to surpass it. He was convinced that the upper cervical x-ray analysis called Blair Analysis, developed by Dr. Bill Blair, D.C. of Texas, was by far the most specific. He began looking for someone who could teach Blair's work, including the stereoscopic x-ray marking. While he never got to see his idea come to fruition, he set the wheels in motion and eventually the system was taught by a very competent Sherman grad, Dr. Perry Rush, who had studied under Blair and Dr. Muncie in California.

The other major focus of the ADIO curriculum was the philosophy and Reggie was the foundation of that department. He taught Philosophy 801. Students, no matter what their background or knowledge of chiropractic, were mesmerized by his class. He would come into class with only a roll book, take roll, put a foot up on a chair and proceed to casually lecture for fifty minutes. His classroom lecture style was almost identical to his speaking style in front of large groups. He speaks smoothly, never faltering or seeming to be at a loss for words. He almost seems to have thousands of 3 x 5 cards filed in his head which his mind flips over as he speaks. He never seems to miss a point, or if he does, he will come back to it so effortlessly and insert it so easily into his presentation that no one could possibly know that it is not the usual order of presentation. It is easy to write off Reggie's ability by the fact that he has lectured to so many classes for so many years that his presentation has become flawless. But having listened to and watched the man teach and speak for over thirty years, I do not believe that is the case. He has a number of unique gifts that blend together to form his unique speaking style. It is rare that one person has a combination of such gifts. Great speakers are not necessarily blessed with brilliant minds just as brilliant minds may be unable to articulate their thoughts in a meaningful or interesting way. Reg has both speaking skills and an uncanny ability to use his mental "card file." He does not just have knowledge stored but is able to arrange the cards in an order to make it logical. His ability to "read" his audience and present the material in a simple, yet elegant way is unique. A person will hear the most technical of information made simple. Reg has a unique charisma about him. It is not the flamboyant, preaching style of so many of today's chiropractic speakers, but there is a definite charisma. He has a special speaking style combined with a wealth of information and exceptional ability to access it. There is perhaps no other speaker quite like him in chiropractic.

His greatest ability by far is to put all of the above talents together in such a way that it convinces people to make a commitment to chiropractic, often a lifetime commitment in an unbelievably short amount of time. There are thousands of lay people who after hearing Reg speak for an hour, have committed to lifetime care. Many of these people went on to become chiropractors. Similarly, there are hundreds, perhaps thousands, of chiropractors who have made changes in their professional lives as a result of Reggie's teaching/speaking. The uniqueness of this ability lies with the fact that he captures and brings together the thought process of his audience by way of clear, logical, deductive thinking and as a result, they have made changes in their lives and/or practice. They may feel that Reg gave them the information but that they actually put it together. Some speakers in chiropractic can emotionally stimulate you by their dynamic presentation and motivate you toward some type of commitment (often it is to give money to some chiropractic cause). However, the next day, when your logical mind kicks in and the emotion is gone, it may not seem like such a good idea. People do not feel that way when Reggie speaks. It is just as sound and logical an idea the next day. Instead of dragging you to an idea by stirring your emotions, he gives you the "directions" so that you can find your way there yourself.

This is not to suggest that every student or chiropractor that hears Reggie present the straight chiropractic philosophy becomes a straight chiropractor for life and never strays from the straight philosophy. To suggest that would be ludicrous. I would venture to say, however, that there are very few who gave up straight chiropractic because it stopped making sense. Some may quit it because they want to practice medicine or therapeutics or because they want to make more money, but not one chiropractor could ever renounce Reggie Gold's idea of straight chiropractic because it no longer made sense. Reg presents the straight chiropractic philosophy in a way that no one before him has been able to and maybe no one will again. There are precious few people in the world who have the unique combination of gifts that Reggie has and rarely do you find one in a profession or in a position within a profession to affect people in such an enormous way. Those that have learned their philosophy from Reggie are truly a fortunate group of people. It has stayed with them because of his unique style that indelibly impacts it upon one's logical mind. Many have chosen to ignore their logical mind and so practice in spite of his teaching but they do not lose it.

Students were getting a good education in philosophy and in technique at ADIO, but the program suffered from outside pressures. It was clear that the ultimate goal of federal recognition for an accrediting agency (SCASA) that would serve the needs of the two straight schools was a long way off. This was not necessarily a function of poor leadership but rather the imposing process of legitimizing an accrediting agency. Further, it was costing money. The more SCASA developed, the more its expenses grew - printing costs, staffing and by now it was reaching the point of needing the expert input of professional educators who had to be paid. SCASA became one more liability to the straight chiropractic community, another drain of its precious few financial resources. It seemed like every week straight chiropractors were being asked to donate to SCASA, Sherman or ADIO. Of course, Sherman was the most established institution of the three and so it received the greatest share. Most chiropractors who wanted to donate their hard earned money preferred to give it to an already proven winner. Sherman had demonstrated that it could graduate students and that they could get into a dozen or so states. They did not have the same confidence in SCASA or ADIO.

By this time, the mixing element of the profession was mobilizing its energies. The National Board of Chiropractic Examiners (NBCE) passed a ruling saying that a college had to be a degree-granting institution for its students to qualify for the exams. ADIO had still not been able to raise the $500,000 required for application to the Pennsylvania State Department of Education. Founders of the school, those who gave $8,000 or more, $5,000 of which was to go to the endowment fund for degree granting status, were trickling in slowly. The money just was not out there and even a great fund raiser like Reggie could not get blood out of a stone. While the school had no financial problems (it was paying its bills and had money in the bank), it was not moving towards the half-million dollar endowment fund needed for degree-granting status. The inability of the students to take the National Boards quickly became a concern. Sherman was not in the same situation inasmuch as the degree-granting status in South Carolina was different than Pennsylvania. It was solely an ADIO problem. Students were getting a little nervous because they would not be able to take the Boards when students from other schools did. These fears were well-founded. As it turned out, many could not take Part I of NBCE exam until they graduated, two years behind other students. This concern caused some to transfer to other schools but there were still many coming in to replace them and the enrollment continued to grow. The State board was still dragging its feet in telling ADIO what it needed to do to get state approval. This was at least partially due to animosity on the part of some of the board members and simple inexperience on the part of others. After Reggie's initial application had not been acted upon for a year, Reg began to get more aggressive, to the point of threatening legal action against the State board. Through constant written communication, he had become familiar with the attorney for the State board and even she was sympathetic to the school's plight. She tried to push the Board to act but as their legal representative she could do little more than encourage the Board to act fairly toward the school.

One of the highlights of the first year was the fall Lyceum in 1978. Until ADIO began , Sherman had been holding two Lyceums a year to provide a semi-annual gathering for the straight chiropractic community. With the opening of ADIO, they graciously agreed to hold one Lyceum in the spring and ADIO would hold its Lyceum in the fall. Sherman still continues the traditional spring Lyceum during Memorial Day Weekend and it is still the most popular gathering of the straight chiropractic community. During ADIO's first Lyceum, many outstanding speakers as well as the school's faculty spoke. Reg ran a fund raising event, and for the students who by that time numbered about seventy-five, the entire Lyceum was a great experience. Reg and the Board of Trustees of ADIO decided to give honorary degrees to Thom Gelardi and Monroe Schneier, D.C., the legislative representative for the Pennsylvania Chiropractic Fellowship. When the news of this honor was made public, the Pennsylvania Department of Education sent the school a letter

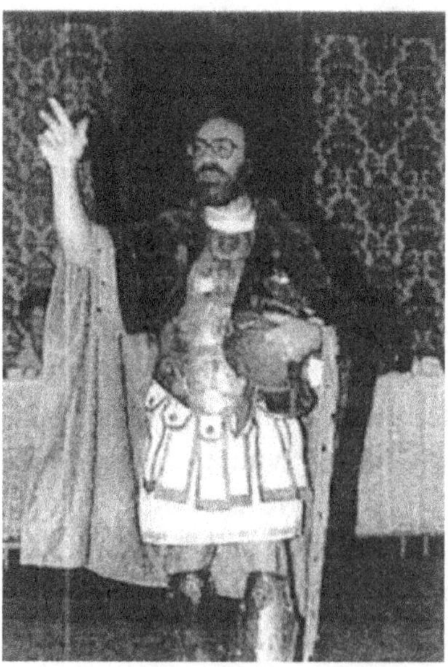

Joe Flesia as a Roman soldier gave an impassioned speech at ADIO's first Lyceum

informing them that since they were not a degree-granting institution, they could not even give honorary degrees. This was an indication of the pressure, the scrutiny and the opposition that the school was constantly subjected to.

The following account represents a serious and unfortunate break in my and Reggie's relationship that lasted for almost five years. While it is personally difficult for me to recount the events that precipitated Reggie's leaving the straight chiropractic movement for a number of years, it nevertheless has historical significance. In fact, perhaps a much greater good came from his subsequent time in Spinology. Be that as it may, we will never know what great things might have happened had Reggie not left ADIO or the straight chiropractic community for that extended period.

When Reggie established ADIO, he wanted to insure that he could control the institution, which was not unusual. Others before him had done it and it was really a matter of common sense. When Palmer College changed to a non-profit organization, B.J. organized the Board of Trustees in such a manner that he could control them. Thom Gelardi did a similar thing at Sherman and Reggie followed suit at ADIO. Chiropractic history is full of incidents where changes and compromises completely transformed an organization as the founder stood helplessly by. Many founders of associations or schools or some other chiropractic institution found their organization changed into the exact opposite of what it was intended to be while they stood by, unable to prevent it because of the structure or the composition of the board of trustees. Reggie was determined that whatever he invested his life and energy into would not go that way. Consequently, he structured the Board of ADIO so that he could control it, having his relatives and close chiropractic associates in position to support him should the need ever arise.

By the Spring of 1979, difficulties were developing that would eventually precipitate Reggie's leaving the school. Reggie was adamant about his idea of not paying a faculty despite the fact that some in the school felt that ADIO was in a position to afford to give instructors some compensation. There is no doubt it would have further hindered the school's raising the needed half million dollars for degree granting status. To Reg, however, it was a matter of principle. In his opinion, instructors made their living in practice and gave back to the profession by teaching. He had never taken salary for teaching at Columbia or his teaching duties at Sherman. His salary at Sherman was strictly for his administrative duties. Nevertheless, by the end of the first year, this policy was taking its toll. Tedd Koren was the first faculty member to leave, actually during the first year. Tedd was beginning to develop some entrepreneurial ideas which would later become Koren Publications and teaching was a drain on his time. After the first year, others began to follow. As mentioned earlier, teaching is a time consuming job. Faculty were coming to school five days a week. All of them except myself were new practitioners and two, Claude Lessard and Ben Tanner, had families. Building a practice is also a full-time job and many faculty members found that their teaching was interfering with that. I personally noticed a drop in my practice as I no longer had the time to do practice-promoting activities. Instead of writing articles for my patients, I was developing lectures for my students. Rather than going out to speak in the community, I was going to classes. Instead of writing ads, I was marking exams. All of the faculty were affected, some more than others. Ultimately, the school was unable to attract faculty because young practitioners realized there was no compensation for teaching.

Of course, with the enrollments rising and new courses being added each quarter, there was a need for more and more faculty. A few local chiropractors came in to help out but Reg solved the problem by hiring administrators who assumed full-time teaching loads. This seemed like a logical and acceptable policy to Reg. The administrators, particularly Academic Dean and Administrative Dean, were not in practice so they deserved to be paid for their full-time work as administrators, just as Reg received a salary as President. By this time, he was teaching two or three classes a day and, of course, was not practicing. Unfortunately, the faculty saw it differently. All they could see was that an administrator taught three hours a day and worked another five and was paid for eight where they taught one, two or three hours a day for nothing and then had to go home and practice for "eight hours" to make a living. The bottom line to them was that someone was being paid for the exact same thing that they were not being paid for. Further, they argued that the idea of having successful practicing chiropractors in teaching positions was not coming to bear because more and more classes were being taught by non-practicing administrators. Both sides had their points but an impasse was clearly approaching. It should not be made to seem that Reggie was exacting slave-labor from the faculty-chiropractors. They were able to apply their "salary" toward becoming a founder and a number of them became founders as a result of teaching. In their defense, they were not mercenary, it was just that, like many, they had made great sacrifices to get through chiropractic college and were expecting to see at least some financial reward.

The conflict eventually came to a crisis. Whether it would have happened without my personal input is debatable, but my presence at the school most definitely brought it to a head. At the time, I occupied two conflicting positions at the college as a faculty member and vice chairman of the Board of Trustees. In a real sense, I was both Reggie's employee (albeit unpaid) and one of his bosses (Trustee status). This placed me in a very uncomfortable position. However, it was my choice to occupy them both. More importantly, it placed Reggie in the very unfavorable position of having a direct line from the faculty to the Trustee Board. When I had a problem as a faculty member, it was not necessary to go through any of the "proper channels" (e.g., faculty committees, faculty chair, etc.). I had a direct conduit to the Board of Trustees, being the vice-chairman. This problem was further compounded by the fact that

Reggie is not an organizational person. Like B.J. and most other great chiropractors, he tends to be autocratic. You could go to him with a problem, any problem, his door was always open, but he was not terribly amenable to dealing with committees or groups. He wanted to handle people on a one-to-one basis, he and his protagonist. 1, along with others, felt uncomfortable in that position primarily because of the awe we had for the man and his persuasive abilities.

It took me a few years but I realize now that I wronged Reggie. Had I just been a member of the Board of Trustees, I would probably not have been involved with the administrative problems between the non-paid faculty and Reggie. On the other hand, had I been merely a faculty member, I would have persevered with the conditions as they were or if I felt I could not continue under the circumstances, I would have quietly resigned my position and gone back to strictly private practice. It was Reggie's school. It could not have begun without him and further, it would not have continued or grown without his leadership. The idea of subjection to Reg's absolute authority and allowing him to either succeed or fail in the school was a new concept to many of us young practitioners. It was supposed that the Board of Trustees ran the school. One faculty member (myself) and one student (John Gallagher) were members of the Board. Further, chiropractors as a whole seem to have difficulties being organizational people. Perhaps it has to do with the individuality aspect of our philosophy and the type of people attracted to chiropractic. In any event, there was a lack of cohesiveness among the administration and faculty. When the issue of paying the faculty came before the Board of Trustees, the members were divided. Some of the Board members were friends and colleagues of the unpaid faculty and others, as mentioned earlier, were loyal to and even related to Reg. The majority was not on Reg's side, however, the way the Board was constructed, Reggie had control. The members that elected (or fired) Board members were those who were loyal to Reg. At one meeting, Reggie let the rest of the Board know that he could replace all of us with new board members. It was his school. However, he also realized that if he did not have the cooperation of the Board and of the faculty, he did not want to continue as the head of ADIO. Reg admits that it was a very negative experience in his life, and to keep the school and be surrounded by the negativism was not worth it to him either professionally or personally. He realized that if he stayed he would have to get many new people both on the Board of Trustees and the faculty and there were not that many good people in the straight chiropractic community. So he chose to resign and to relinquish control of the school. He did not know what would happen to it but he was confident that it was in good hands philosophically, which is quite a compliment to myself and the others who took over the school. So in early August of 1979, at a specially called meeting of the Board of Trustees, Reggie resigned his position as President of ADIO Institute of Straight Chiropractic, a position he had held for just over two years. Irene had shortly before that left Sherman for the purpose of becoming the Director of ADIO's Health Center (i.e., Clinic) which was to open in the fall of 1979. She was also going to teach morning classes. Irene, of course, resigned with Reggie as did P.J. Martin and two administrators, Walt Giddings, D.C. who had come from Indiana to be Administrative Dean, and Chris Kent, D.C., a former faculty member from Palmer College who had arrived only a few days before to be the Academic Dean.

To a great many people's surprise, ADIO continued to function without Reg and even prospered. Many of the school's problems were still unresolved when Reg left, most of which were the result of outside opposition and would have been there whether or not Reg was President. He left the school in good financial condition, partly because of good fiscal judgment and partly because of having an inexpensive faculty for twenty months. Most importantly, Reggie left the school in the hands of people that were still committed to his philosophy. Whatever the feelings that developed between Reggie and the core of people that opposed him and eventually controlled the school, they still recognized the philosophy that he had given to them and the importance of the school in preserving and perpetuating that philosophy. That love for Reg's philosophy did not leave with him. ADIO continued for more than sixteen years after Reggie left it, eventually gaining degree-granting status and changing its name to Pennsylvania College of Straight Chiropractic. It continued to teach the philosophy that Reg had given to it at its inception until the last year or so. Many believe that it was the compromise of that philosophy that led to the school's eventual closing. While Reggie's two years at ADIO left him with mixed feelings and broken friendships, some of which have yet to be "repaired," the school made a great contribution to the straight chiropractic movement. Hundreds of straight chiropractors are in practice today as a result of their education under Reggie and those who continued to teach his straight chiropractic philosophy. His impact upon the school's graduates will continue for many years to come.

It is sad that the faculty salary issue could not have been resolved without the break that took place. It might have become a moot point in future years. Dr. Warren Evans from the Pennsylvania Department of Education stated about a year and a half after the incident that not paying faculty would have been unacceptable to his department for a school seeking degree-granting status. Further, accreditation people also said that the salary status of a faculty was an important factor in gaining accreditation. Yet, in the latter years of Penn Straight (ADIO), Reggie's concerns about paying faculty became clear. Many of the faculty then were dependent upon the school for their salaries and practice was a sideline if anything at all. Many of them were not the role model of a successful straight chiropractor to the students at the college. Many who were not adequate as straight chiropractors even denigrated the straight philosophy and practice and detracted from the objective of the school. Reg apparently was able to foresee this problem occurring and that is why he took such a strong unyielding stand. To Reg, it was a matter of principle and he could not and would not compromise on principle. To a number of good straight chiropractors it was not a matter of principle but of opinion and Reg's unwillingness to yield to the majority opinion was the unfortunate basis for a split. The day Reg left ADIO was a sad day for the straight chiropractic movement for when he left the school he also left straight chiropractic and immediately turned his attention toward a new profession, Spinology.

CHAPTER 5

Spinology

1980 -1986

Less than four months after leaving ADIO, Reggie launched his next project, the development of Spinology. The first school opened in Philadelphia in January, 1980. Reggie was previously nurturing the idea in his mind, for even he could not have put together the Spinology program in just three months. In actuality, Reggie has always seen the Spinology model as the ultimate in a chiropractic education and practice. But long before he was even born, the chiropractic profession had embarked upon the licensure road. State regulation, rather than the philosophy and objective, dictated to the profession what its educational program should be. Joseph Keating, in his book review of *Refined by Fire: The Evolution of Straight Chiropractic*, stated that straight chiropractic was an outgrowth of Spinology. Reggie's idea for Spinology, however, existed before the fall of 1979 as straight chiropractic. The profession had just not had the luxury of describing straight chiropractic without all the medical baggage. It still does not fully enjoy that luxury. Reggie was able to do that with Spinology. Reg himself maintains that if B.J. were alive today, he would be right where Spinology was in 1980 and where straight chiropractic is today. Many of the courses at all of the chiropractic schools, including Sherman and ADIO, were license driven and taught simply to obtain or maintain "governmental (state board) recognition." It was understood that this would not change unless or until the state laws changed.

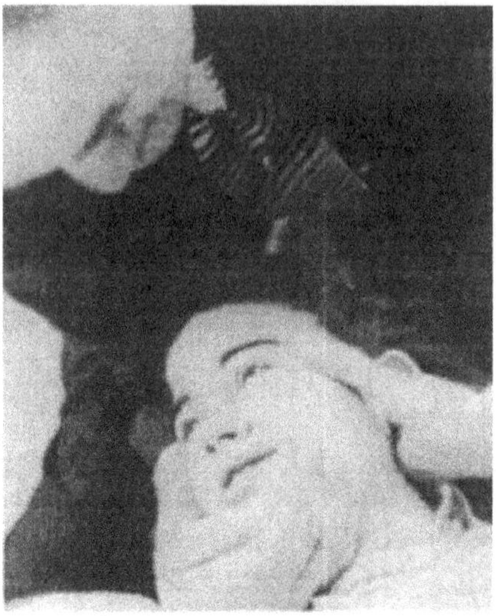

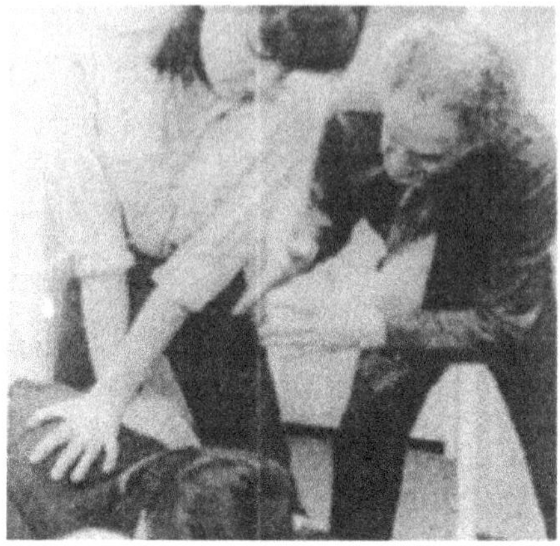

Small classes, personal demonstration and individual instruction result in confident and competent spinologiests.

Spinal Tutorium Catalog, page 13

When Reg left ADIO, he was, for the first time, totally unfettered to design chiropractic the way it should have been, the way he believed it was meant to be. It was as if he were given the chiropractic philosophy and a clean white page. He could draw up the plans for his model of chiropractic any way he wanted with only one restriction - he could not call it chiropractic! Once he was able to get past that obstacle, it was clear sailing. And for Reg, that was not really difficult. He had grown out of the HIO technique associated with B.J. He had renounced his allegiance to Palmer by his involvement with Sherman and then ADIO. He had split with traditional chiropractic in moving from a non-therapeutic model and in resigning from the ICA. He had even, for all practical purposes, relinquished the title of doctor and had been known simply as Reggie for many years. The stage was set for his model of chiropractic and Spinology was as good a name as any for it. The big question of course was, how ready was the rest of the world. The mixing aspect of the profession was not at all ready. The straight chiropractic community, including those who had followed and supported Reg over the years had mixed emotions. Reggie had thought that the straight community would see the wisdom of what to him was a logical progression for straight chiropractic and that they would support his efforts. Some did, many did not. What Reg perhaps underestimated was the pride of many in the straight chiropractic profession and how their ego would stand in the way of taking chiropractic to its next level of service to humanity. The two manifestations of that pride, the issue of licensure and the right to be called doctor were the two that Spinology would of necessity have to relinquish. They were two things even most straights actively took pride in and simply were not ready to give up.

Licensing has always been a two-edged sword. While it gave some degree of legitimacy, it was also restrictive. It forced the licensee to abide by the dictates of a government agency. In the case of chiropractic, it was often the mixing aspect of the profession with the weight of the state behind them. Licensing has one purpose and it is not to legitimize a profession or to build up its image or acceptance. Licensing is designed to protect the public. When you are providing a service that has the potential to be harmful to the public, then that service and its providers need to be regulated. When chiropractic was in the business of getting sick people well and relating to disease, it needed licensing. A doctor had to be held accountable for his ability to determine whether it was reasonable to expect his care to accomplish its objective or whether the patient should seek help elsewhere. The model of chiropractic that Reg had come to embrace did not relate to disease, its prevention, its cure or its cause. It related to correcting vertebral subluxations so that the human body could work at its maximum potential, free of nerve interference. What's more, the delivery of that service presented no health danger to the public, at least none that warranted government regulation.

The problem with this was that according to many, including chiropractors and the public at large, licensing was a stamp of approval. Our profession had gone to great expense to be licensed and to ask them to give it up when even hairdressers and plumbers had to be licensed was a heavy blow to their collective egos. To further complicate the issue, straight chiropractors were as proud of the title "doctor" as any chiropractor and to ask them to give that up was too much to ask. To accept the Spinology model would require being stripped of your title. This was especially difficult for straight chiropractors who believed that being grounded in the non-diagnostic chiropractic philosophy made them more "learned" and more of an "authority" in the profession and consequently, more deserving of the title "doctor." Reggie's mistake was overestimating the humanitarian inclinations of the straight community and underestimating its pride in its status in the professional community.

As far as the differences between objective straight chiropractic and the practice of Spinology, there are none, at least not according to one practicing straight chiropractor. Dr. Thomas Gregory was a practicing Spinologist before attending and graduating from Pennsylvania College of Straight Chiropractic. He says of Spinology, "It is exactly the same way I practice now." The philosophy differed only in some aspects of the terminology. When Spinology was just beginning, Reg used the term "vertebral subluxation," but later he changed it to "spinal obtrusion." He maintains that the word "subluxation" had so many different meanings that it became meaningless, as a means of describing what the Spinologist addressed. The obtrusion was described by Stephenson's classical four components

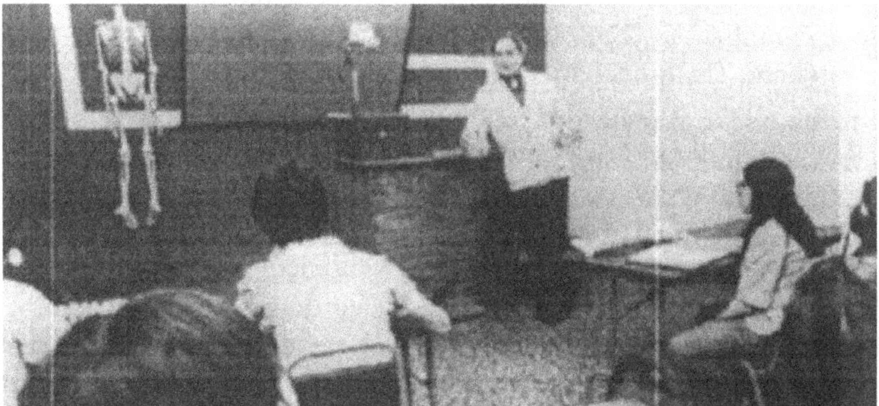

Spinal Tutorium Catalog, page 2

of the vertebral subluxation but by calling it a spinal obtrusion it remained that and only that. When the term "spinal obtrusion" was used, Spinologists knew exactly what they were talking about.

So philosophically, Spinology was incorporated in the chiropractic that Reg had taught before leaving ADIO. The practice was also the same up to the point of addressing symptoms. Reg was leaving the Spinology door open for chiropractors who would be harassed by an increasingly hostile mixer state board trying to force them into doing medical, diagnostic procedures. A few chiropractors took advantage of Reggie's offer and went through the Spinology program or an abbreviated version of it to become certified. Spinology allowed Reg to teach and practice objective straight chiropractic at the next level. Straight chiropractic was still a "health profession" and until he got into Spinology, Reg could not break away from that. It is true that addressing human potential was related to health in the broadest definition of the term. Joe Flesia and Guy Riekeman had given the straight chiropractic community a broad definition and it satisfied most straight chiropractors. However, while the straights defined health as "physical, mental and social well-being and not merely the absence of symptoms and disease," the majority of the public associated health with disease and medical problems. Straight chiropractic had (and still has) that stigma. Spinology was free of it.

Reg always believed that chiropractic was too good for most chiropractors while their pride in their increasingly medical education and their degrees had caused chiropractors to think they were better than chiropractic. Spinology resolved that problem. As a Spinologist, you could not treat medical conditions, you could not diagnose and you could not call yourself a doctor. Everything you did and said focused on the person and the philosophy. You could not take credit as the healer or the doctor. In fact, if anyone offered to treat or cure anything, they would lose their standing as a Spinologist and perhaps risk arrest for violating a state statute, relating to the practice of medicine, chiropractic or both. Reg felt that straight chiropractic was doomed, despite the dedicated efforts on the part of many people who wanted it to succeed. He believed that the opposition was too great and the cost more than the straight profession was able or willing to pay. The cost of keeping ADIO and Sherman alive was astronomical. Hundreds of thousands of dollars a year were being spent in legal fees alone. The cost of maintaining SCASA and trying to see it achieve recognition by the Department of Education was tremendous. At this time, the two schools were almost totally tuition driven, enrollments were not growing to meet the financial needs and the few donations that were coming in were from the same individuals who were just about tapped out. Without the schools, almost everyone believed that the straight chiropractic movement would die. Spinology was the escape hatch for the thousands of chiropractors whose only desire was to correct vertebral subluxations to allow the innate intelligence of the body to be better expressed.

Reg himself makes the differentiation between Spinology and straight chiropractic in that while straight chiropractic may address itself to health and human potential, Spinology addressed only human potential. He maintains that health is only 5% of the human experience and only 5% of what the correction of vertebral subluxation by a chiropractor addresses. Spinology addressed the other 95%. Most straight chiropractors address only the 5%. The majority of the patients coming into a straight chiropractic office are, at best, interested in having their health restored or maintained. Despite the efforts of straight chiropractors to educate their patients, they are still often viewed as health professionals. The patients may understand that the straight chiropractor is not treating their disease or medical condition but instead comes to have the vertebral subluxation component of their health addressed. Straight chiropractors have tried to expand the definition of health to include all areas of performance potential and a number of chiropractors have been very good at articulating this expanded definition of health. Unfortunately, the general population still views the straight chiropractor as a health-care professional. As a spinologist, you are not allowed to talk about health, not even to relate the correction of spinal obtrusions to that "5%" of a person's performance. The Spinologist is limited to the other 95%.

Reggie's goal was to have thousands of Spinology schools across the world, to supply the need for every man, woman and child on

GENERAL INFORMATION

LOCATIONS:	Philadelphia Spinal Tutorium 7151 Frankford Avenue Philadelphia, Pennsylvania 19135	San Francisco Tutorium 2200 Central Avenue Alameda, California 94501	
DURATION OF COURSE:	One Year (3 trimesters of 12 weeks each)		
ENROLLMENTS:	New enrollments are accepted at the beginning of each trimester		
CALENDAR OF TRIMESTER DATES:	**1984**	**1985**	**1986**
	Jan. 9 - Mar. 30 Apr. 9 - June. 29 Sep. 4 - Nov. 21	Jan. 7 - Mar. 29 Apr. 9 - Jun. 28 Sep. 3 - Nov. 22	Jan. 6 - Mar. 28 Apr. 7 - Jun. 27 Sep. 8 - Nov. 28
COURSE HOURS:	Choice of 9:00 am to 1:00 pm or 6:00 pm to 10:00 pm		

SUBJECTS:		
	Philosophy and Doctrine	60 hours
	Spinology Technique	180 hours
	Innate Matter	60 hours
	Communications	120 hours
	Business Procedures	60 hours
	Practice Management	30 hours
	Practical Experience	240 hours

PREREQUISITES FOR ADMISSION:	To enroll you must: be at least 18 years of age. be proficient in the English language, and demonstrate sufficient physical and mental ability to complete the course satisfactorily.
TUITION FEES:	$3000.00 total. Payable in advance or in three $1000.00 installments at the beginning of each trimester or in thirty weekly payments of $105.00 each. N.B. In the installment system, the additional $5.00 per installment is a bookkeeping fee which amounts to 16.75%, and brings the total cost to $3150.00 N.B. The information contained herein is dated and subject to change without notice.
FOR FURTHER INFORMATION, WRITE OR PHONE:	Philadelphia Spinal Tutorium 7151 Frankford Avenue Philadelphia, Pennsylvania 19135 (215) 624-8700

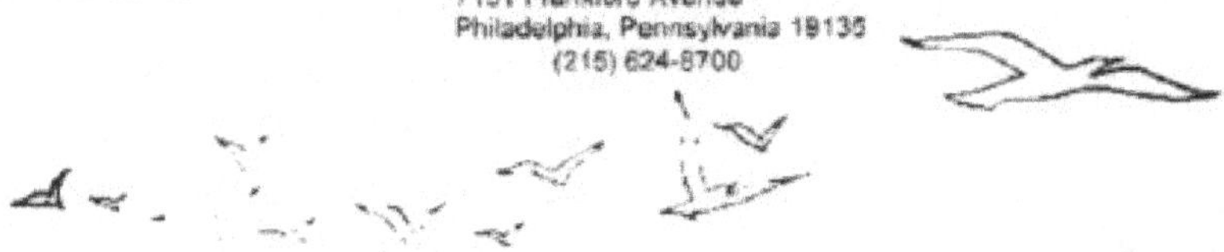

Spinal Tutorium Catalog, pages 19 and 20

the face of the earth to have their spines checked on a regular basis. At first thought, the idea seems to be preposterous, thousands of Spinology schools when we barely have twenty chiropractic schools worldwide. But on further reflection the idea of thousands of Spinology schools is not preposterous, the reality of only twenty chiropractic schools is. If we truly believe that chiropractic is good for improving potential in every area of life and we believe that all of humanity should have it available to them, then the idea of taking so few chiropractors into the profession is a travesty. Of course the majority of the profession does not have this perception of chiropractic, but even the straight chiropractic segment of the profession has no plans for new schools and the only remaining straight school has publicly announced that it is limiting its enrollment. That may be great to provide an attractive faculty/student ratio, but it does not solve the problem of having billions of human beings live and die without ever having received even one chiropractic adjustment. Regardless of your feelings about Spinology, you have to admit that Reggie had a vision of "adjustments for the world" that the straight chiropractic community has apparently forsaken. Even Sid Williams, who at one time had a similar vision for chiropractic, appears to have abandoned that idea. The growth of his schools has leveled off in the last few years and he has put his energies and money into building athletic facilities.

During the six years of Reg's involvement with Spinology, he opened four Spinology Tutoriums. The first was in Philadelphia, then he opened others in San Francisco, Spain and South America. There were plans for one in Hong Kong, but it never materialized. Reggie was convinced as were many others, that the chiropractic profession was and still is practicing "birth control." Chiropractic continues to be in a unique position. There are not enough chiropractors to create universal acceptance but there are too many to support the profession with the musculoskeletal model that the profession is currently perpetuating. We should either drastically limit the number of "bad back doctors" going into practice or develop a different model for chiropractic. Almost everyone in the profession realizes this dilemma. The accrediting agency and state boards want to limit the profession rather than accept a model that could be applied to all human beings. Increased pre-requisite requirements, additional parts to licensing exams, more and more accreditation requirements which raise the cost of chiropractic education may be done to raise the respect for the chiropractor in the eyes of the health care community but it also serves to limit those entering chiropractic college. Apparently, most of the profession is willing to go along with this professional birth control by not opposing the above actions. Spinology was simply an objection to that action.

Those who studied and practiced Spinology had a strong commitment to the non-therapeutic approach, more so even than most graduates from straight chiropractic colleges. They did not have the tradition of getting sick people well that straight chiropractic had to contend with. They were not doctors. In fact, the few who were also doctors of chiropractic, who for one reason or another could not or did not want to practice chiropractic, were forbidden to call themselves doctor in their Spinology practice. Unlike the straight chiropractic student, they were not inundated with medical education. In fact, there were no Pathology or Diagnosis courses taught at the Spinology Tutorium. The education was confined to Philosophy, Practice Building, Communications, and a small amount of Anatomy and Physiology to understand the spine and appreciate the beauty of the body's innate intelligence and, of course, adjusting courses. Reggie taught the philosophy, communications and business procedures courses. In the beginning P.J. Martin, a former ADIO faculty member, and Glenn Allen, a former ADIO student who had both left the chiropractic school when Reggie did, taught technique. As Spinologists graduated, some of the more proficient ones stayed on to help teach. Occasionally Irene would come to help teach. This very focused education helped keep Spinology students from being tainted with the therapeutic model as were most chiropractic college graduates. Last but not least, Spinology graduates did not have to cope with fellow practitioners who were doing anything and everything and calling it Spinology. Straight chiropractic college graduates were not so fortunate. On a few occasions, when Reggie learned of Spinologists doing something other than correcting obtrusions, he threatened to withdraw their certification and to take legal action if necessary. Reggie controlled the word "Spinologist," copyrighted it as a trademark, so an individual could not call himself or herself a Spinologist without his certification. A warning was usually enough to get the Spinologist back in line. Reggie made it clear that if the Spinologist was practicing any form of therapeutic procedure, that he would have no reservations about turning the violation into the State Medical Board or Chiropractic Board or both. Although there was no licensing of a Spinologist, Reggie had control of the practice of Spinology through this mechanism.

When the San Francisco Spinology Tutorium began, it was run by P.J. Martin and Mike Dobbins. P.J. was actually the first practicing Spinologist, opening her office in September 1980. P.J. had a chiropractic practice from the time she came to Pennsylvania from South Carolina to teach at ADIO. She changed it into a Spinology practice. The Spain school was run by Michelle and Miguel Bolufer. They were also Sherman graduates and had been running a successful chiropractic practice in Spain. They were long-time friends of Reggie and Irene's and over the years had caught a glimpse of Reggie's vision for Spinology and were anxious to help. Although they ran the school, Reg was often there to help them.

The Spinology program consisted of three, 12-week trimesters. The cost was $1,000 per trimester. Classes were limited to fifteen students, although a night class was occasionally instituted when enrollment was greater than fifteen. Some simple mathematics shows that the Tutorium was grossing less than $1300 a week (15 students x $1,000 / 12 weeks). It is clear that the schools were not profitable. In fact, right up to the end, Spinology required Reggie's own personal funds to exist. Each day of the first trimester consisted of an hour of philosophy, two hours of technique and an hour of basic anatomy and physiology. Someone in the chiropractic profession once asked Reggie why the Spinology student did not learn the physiology of digestion. Reggie replied, "The innate intelligence of the body knows how to do it, why does the Spinology student have to learn it also?" Each day of the second trimester consisted of one hour of communications, two hours of technique and one hour of practice building. The third trimester was almost entirely practical in nature. The Spinology student would literally build a Spinology practice at the Tutorium, including bringing people in, doing an orientation with them and adjusting them.

There is an interesting but little known aspect of Spinology that perhaps if known would have lessened the antagonism toward it by some members of the chiropractic profession. About half of the students in the Philadelphia Tutorium and virtually all of the students in the Tutoriums outside the United States were not Americans. We, in the straight community, always talk about chiropractic for the world and how important it is for all people to have their spines checked on a regular basis. Even the "subluxation based" chiropractor, who represents a majority of the profession, agrees with the need for adjustments and "promoting a vertebral subluxation-free world." Through Spinology, Reg was providing an opportunity for millions of people to have their spines checked and adjusted, people who would probably never even hear of chiropractic. The likelihood that chiropractic would have an impact on any third-world country is not great. Spinologists, however, could go back to their countries, to their cities and their villages and adjust the spines of their people. Those people would not care whether the person adjusting them had two years of pre-professional training, a diploma from an accredited chiropractic college, a license or anything else. What's more, by not calling it chiropractic in foreign countries, it would not reflect upon chiropractic (although the good they would do could only have had a positive reflection). Spinology was clearly no threat to chiropractic. With the cost of chiropractic education, the time involved, the expense of coming from a foreign country and the unavailability of student loans for foreign students, the likelihood of many third world countries ever sending nationals to chiropractic college was and remains remote. The fact that there are very few people entering the profession with the heart of Mother Teresa means that we are not going to see many American students heading off to the jungles or the Calcutta slums to adjust the people. We are fortunate in this country that there are very few people who cannot find someone to adjust them if they want to. Spinology could have provided that opportunity for the rest of the world with an unlicensed, non-doctor profession. Reg had traveled all over the world, promoting Spinology for the six years that he was involved in it. Had it caught on, it could have been a tremendous boon to mankind. We in the chiropractic profession boasted in our centennial celebration what a blessing chiropractic has been to humanity. Yet, the U.S. represents less than 5% of the world's population and less than 20% of people in the U.S. go to a chiropractor. Perhaps less than one tenth of 1% receive regular care. Spinology could have made a tremendous difference.

Perhaps the greatest contribution to be made by Reggie's development of Spinology was given to the straight chiropractic profession. Spinology was always Reggie's ideal for chiropractic. His development of the philosophy and practice during this period away from the chiropractic profession was unencumbered by curriculum, accreditation, restrictive licensing exams, state boards or "doctor" titles. He did not have to think about how his new model of adjusting subluxations would be accepted or how it would fit into the present models of chiropractic. That had to be a tremendously freeing experience for him in his thinking. Whether it was worth the pain that he felt in leaving ADIO and the chiropractic profession only he can say. I believe from the straight chiropractic profession's viewpoint, that hiatus was good. It enabled straight chiropractic's greatest thinker to tighten, develop and further simplify the philosophy that would be straight chiropractic in the 90's.

While Reg was turning out Spinologists between 1980 and 1987 there were chiropractors who for various reasons wanted to become Spinologists. A few saw Reggie's vision and wanted to be part of it. Others could not get a chiropractic license for one reason or another and approached Reggie for the right to practice Spinology. He made it clear that they could not call themselves a doctor even if they had received a D.C. degree from a chiropractic college. They could not associate themselves with chiropractic, they could not do any of the things associated with non-straight chiropractic like diagnosis or treat disease and they could not do some of the things associated with straight chiropractic, such as x-ray. Reggie had copyrighted the words "Spinology" and "Spinologist" and to use the title necessitated being certified through him. Of course, any activities that were not in keeping with that of a Spinologist, namely mixing, put a practitioner in danger of losing his or her certification and, more importantly, the right to call what they were doing Spinology. Reggie realized that one of the great downfalls of D.D. and B.J.'s chiropractic was that they had no control over the practitioners and today not only do those distorting the original tenets of chiropractic outnumber the adherents but they also control most state boards and the accrediting agency. Reggie was determined that this would not happen to Spinology. The long range goals of Spinology were carefully planned out and assurance of Spinology's continued existence was protected. Reg accomplished this by starting the Church of the Triune, which protected the rights of Spinologists under the Freedom of Religion Amendment of the United States Constitution.

The idea of giving chiropractic a quasi-religious status was not new. D.D. suggested it in his posthumously published 1914 book, *The Chiropractor.* George Shears, D.C., the founder of the G.P.C. (God-Patient-Chiropractor) Fee System, also suggested it as an alternative to licensing laws. B.J. always rejected the idea. Many in the profession were very critical of Reggie for this idea, saying he was trying to turn chiropractic into a religion under the guise of Spinology. It is very interesting that most of the people that were critical of Reg for giving Spinology a religious status (something it never had to use), have no problem adding the rituals of medicine as well as its terminology to chiropractic so that we can "survive." Making chiropractic into medicine is just as abhorrent an idea as making it or Spinology a religion. Reg had no desire to make Spinology a religion but he wanted to assure its continued existence. Today, Reg admits that making it a religion was a mistake and was not necessary.

HUMAN POTENTIAL

The magnitude of human potential will never be fully understood. It defies imagination, for imagination itself is but one small expression of the very potential it would seek to envision. Certainly, human potential is multifaceted. To even begin to appreciate it, one would have to consider such manifestations as:

- The ability to adapt to an ever-changing environment, agreed by most biologists to be the essence of life itself.
- The ability to convert food into walking, talking, flesh and blood.
- The ability to manufacture and balance, in perfect quantity and quality: insulin, cortizone, adrenalin, and every other hormone, enzyme and chemical needed for normal life.
- The ability to reproduce.
- The ability to resist and prevent disease.
- The ability to recover from disease and to repair injury.
- The ability to engage in creative thought and analysis.
- The ability to compose music, prose, and poetry.
- The ability to draw, paint and sculpt.
- The ability to adapt to emotional stress and to develop appropriate emotional responses.
- The ability to remember some things while relegating others to the "inactive" file.
- The ability to maintain balance and to simultaneously coordinated a multitude of different muscular skills for work or play.
- The ability to study and learn.
- The ability to add, subtract, multiply and divide.
- The ability to solve problems and to organize.
- The ability to make decisions.
- The ability to love and trust.
- The ability to accept and respond to the spoken and unspoken needs of others and to share the responsibility for the shaping of our world.
- The ability to shut off conscious thought, to relax and meditate or sleep.

These are but a few of the tangible and intangible expressions of human potential. What a tragedy it is for any part of this potential to be unfulfilled.

In a society committed to specialization, we tend to lose sight of the fact that all of these potentials must interact together in harmony if any are to reach their full expression. The human begin is not a collection of disrelated parts, but an integrated whole with each facet dependent on every other.

The communication and control system (brain, spinal cord, nerves and chemical messengers) coordinate and run the entire human being. damage to this control system must inevitably result in failure of the parts to interact properly. This, in turn, causes a lessening of the ability to express full potential in both tangible and intangible manifestations.

Spinologists are committed to unleashing full potential by maintaining the integrity of the body's control and communication system.

Human Potential is just too valuable to be wasted

Spinal Tutorium Catalog, page 23

Fie had been influenced by others to do it. His only desire was to keep the government's hand off Spinology. However, by not dealing with health or disease in any way, there was no need for it. Spinology was not a danger to anyone and consequently, did not need to be regulated. Most authorities realized that the Spinologist was not a threat to the public welfare. They did not address disease, they did not discourage a person from seeking medical care and they did not present Spinology as an alternative to medical care. Its emphasis on increasing the individual's human potential made Spinology less of a healing art than reflexology, various forms of massage and other therapeutic measures all of which are largely unregulated.

The controlling Triune Church expected its members to begin to contribute 10% of their gross income after the first year in practice. This money would be put toward beginning new Tutoriums all over the world, with a goal of 5,000 eventually. It would also go toward legal battles to protect Spinologists and ultimately a world-wide public relations and advertising campaign. There were a myriad of circumstances affecting the entire movement. For example, the Second Amendment protection was only applicable to the United States. Also, any sort of regulation was unheard of in many third world countries, so Spinologists could legally call themselves chiropractors, except for Reg's vehement opposition. There were very few court cases and none of the few that went to trial were lost by the Spinologists although sometimes the harassment caused the Spinologist to give up practice or go "underground" much like some chiropractors in the early days.

Not only was there virtually no opposition from the authorities, but there was also none from the chiropractic profession, at least none from a legal standpoint. There were, of course, editorials and written diatribes against Reg and Spinology. These problems were usually the result of jealous chiropractors. The sad commentary is not that these few situations occurred but that the chiropractic profession did not do more. The lack of opposition to Spinology was an acknowledgment by the profession that chiropractic had drifted so far from the original philosophy of the Palmers that practicing chiropractic in its purest and most advanced form, distilling it to the very essence of the Palmer's idea, was totally unrecognizable as chiropractic and therefore, it was not necessary to oppose its unregulated practice. The profession, generally speaking, was moving further and further from the Spinology model so those who were taking the profession in that direction saw no need to even address Spinology. I would imagine, however, if Spinology had become very popular and began to have an economic effect upon chiropractic that the leadership and regulatory agencies would have gone after it. That would have made for some interesting legal and philosophical arguments, something that perhaps the chiropractic profession was afraid of and another reason why Spinology was left alone. Reg had them backed in a comer. If Spinology was chiropractic, why was the average chiropractor learning and practicing something totally different? If Spinology was different, then what business did the chiropractic profession have bothering it? While there was relatively little reaction to Spinology, all of it was overwhelmingly negative. Those of the mixing profession, who never really cared for Reg to begin with, who thought that a straight chiropractor was not a "real doctor" but merely a technician, felt vindicated by Reggie going into Spinology. They had no ability to grasp the idea that being a "real doctor" was not important to a straight chiropractor or to a Spinologist. What was important was what he or she was doing.

Reg caused some friction between himself and even his good friends in chiropractic with Spinology. His allegiance was to Spinology and its practitioners during the years he was involved in it. Consequently, he was often forced to say negative things about chiropractors in trying to explain Spinology. It was not purposeful, it was necessary. Rather than judge him for it, straight chiropractors should realize that historically they have done that with medicine and continue to do it today. In trying to explain the ADIO philosophy of chiropractic, straight chiropractors often point out the shortcomings of the outside-in practice of medicine. Reg had to show that Spinology was different than the chiropractic practiced by 99% of the chiropractors. So to emphasize that, to establish the Spinologist's right to practice without governmental harassment, Reg had to make statements like "chiropractic was directed toward disease and its cause." In many states that is exactly what the law said and most chiropractors practice that way. Unfortunately, a few of the 1% that were not practicing that way were offended by what he said. These chiropractors were the very ones that Reggie had influenced to practice a non-therapeutic approach to chiropractic over the years. Many of them, including myself, understood where he was coming from and felt no personal affront but there were others who saw him attacking the very chiropractors he had helped mold.

What Reg was not prepared for was the response by so-called friends. He received a tremendous amount of vicious hate mail from chiropractors. One seminar/practice management consultant wrote him exceptionally vicious attacks, however, when Reg got back into the straight chiropractic movement, he asked him to speak at one of his seminars. Wes Trout, who was one of the first people to invite Reg on to his program when he was still into Spinology, received a good deal of criticism for having Reg as a speaker. Those people who were his close friends never wrote him and never gave him any encouragement. He really only had contact with Wes, Thom Gelardi, Dick Plummer, Joe Donofrio and maybe a few others throughout the "Spinology period." He received no positive responses with the exception of the above. Reg was unprepared for that. He believed that the straight chiropractors who were with him from the Spring Valley days until Spinology would have grasped his vision and supported his efforts if not with money, at least with encouragement. He got none. While Reg maintains that he does not need other people's support when he is on a crusade that he knows is right, the tremendous silence from the straight chiropractic community had to hurt him. There were a few chiropractors like Walt Giddings, P.J. Martin and Chris Kent and, of course, Irene who were with him at ADIO and followed him into Spinology, but they were the only ones.

The straight community was involved in tremendous legal battles with the CCE and others, and at the time was trying to get recognition for their approach to the practice of chiropractic. They were not happy about Spinology which they thought could be used against them by the mixing aspect of the profession. On the other hand, with the formation of Spinology a new profession was in place that could be a safety valve for straight chiropractors. SCASA was still struggling to develop its standards let alone get approved by the federal government. ADIO was trying to survive, with students who had no assurance of getting a license anywhere and no chance of getting student loans. Sherman was a little better off but not much, and both schools were suing everybody in sight from the Department of Education, to the CCE and the ACA, with no success in any of the suits. For a while it looked like Spinology could be a refuge for straight chiropractors. As it turned out, SCASA was eventually recognized by the federal government and straight chiropractors' best days were yet to come. Unfortunately, that changed as quickly as the Washington administration so that even today it is comforting to many straight chiropractors that there is something in place like Spinology just in case. In fact, just before Sherman became accredited by the CCE in 1996, Reggie and Thom discussed the possibility of Spinology becoming active once again in the event that the CCE did not accredit Sherman College. Fortunately for Sherman and the straight chiropractic movement, that accreditation came through.

Spinology did serve a valuable purpose and continues to even at the time of this writing. There are Spinologists in Bogata, Nicaragua, Lema Peru, as well as Pennsylvania, South Carolina, and Massachusetts. There is a school of Spinology active in Australia. Even with all that present activity, there were a number of reasons why Spinology never took off like Reggie had hoped and fully expected it would. First, it was difficult to get a Spinology practice going because Spinology was unheard of by the general public. It often took at least two years to build even a small practice and many Spinologists could not afford that time. In this way they were in the same boat as many of their straight chiropractic cousins, many of whom turned to mixing and ripping off insurance companies. Spinologists did not have that luxury. Some Spinologists believed that it took a charismatic individual or a great salesperson to succeed right away, someone like Reggie. That is not to say that many Spinologists were not successful, although it is really difficult to determine just how successful any particular Spinologist was. Some wanted to keep their daytime jobs and just wanted to develop small part-time practices for family and a few friends and neighbors. For them, Spinology provided exactly what they wanted. But the opportunity to build a large, successful

Spinology practice was not there for many. Some had come from foreign countries to Philadelphia and had spent the last of their money. While the Spinologist did not have student loans to pay back, he or she also had little access to bank loans to finance the opening of a Spinology practice.

Other Spinologists found it difficult to build a practice in part because of the fee system structure that Reg had devised and insisted upon. The fee was an annual fee rather than a per visit fee. This idea was in keeping with the concept that Spinology care was not like medical or chiropractic "fee for care." It was designed to more closely resemble a health club membership. The "recipient" was expected to pay a yearly fee and had unlimited access to spinal checkups. The thinking was that if the person paid in advance for a year's care, they were more likely to use it and see the benefits of regular care. This is the same system that Reg advocates today for chiropractors. However, for Spinologists to interest people totally unfamiliar with the idea of Spinology into this commitment was more difficult a task than some could handle. Even terminology like "recipient" was difficult for the Spinologist to get across to the public. On one occasion a newspaper article, although favorable to the Tutorium, described the recipients as patients. Reg had to send a letter to the paper asking them to correct it and keep a copy of the registered letter in case they did not print the correction or if a problem arose because patients are associated with health care.

The major reason why Spinology did not succeed as Reggie hoped it would was that Reggie himself abandoned it. He had started Spinology because he truly believed that straight chiropractic was not going to survive. He did not believe that ADIO would make it. In fact, it did not, but somehow managed to hold on longer than many expected. He felt the accreditation problems that faced both schools, plus the opposition from almost every other aspect of the profession, were more than the schools could handle. However, when things began to look better for Sherman and ADIO, by this time the name had been changed to Pennsylvania College of Straight Chiropractic, some in the profession convinced Reg that his impact would be greater if he would rejoin the straight chiropractic community. Those that knew Reg and understood where he was coming from realized that his Spinology model was really the ideal practice of straight chiropractic, so there was little problem in Reg making the transition back to straight chiropractic. Those that had a personal problem with Reggie were not happy with his return and felt he should be permanently banished from straight chiropractic. The rest were overjoyed at the prospects of straight chiropractic's most articulate spokesman and most visionary thinker returning to the profession. For Reg, it was an opportunity to return to his first love. Spinology did not have the rich heritage of chiropractic nor the opportunity for Reg to expose as many people as possible to his philosophy. Chiropractic was a ready made audience. Spinology was an audience that Reggie himself had to go out and get and there was a tremendous opposition to it.

There was one more reason which may have influenced Reg to set aside his active involvement with Spinology and rejoin the straight chiropractic movement. The age-old problem in straight chiropractic was trying to keep people straight when finances and egos tempted them to mix. Reggie felt he had solved the problem with Spinology by controlling the practitioners' right to use the word Spinology. If a Spinologist would deviate from the fine line of Spinology, they would first get a call from Reg and a warning. There were some who did this. One was a Spinologist in the Northeast who was giving out the "Chart of Effects of Spinal Misalignment," published by Parker. He was telling his clients that if they had one of these problems, adjustments could correct it. When Reg found out, he gave him a call. If a call did not stop the Spinologist from his errant practice, Reg would remove his certification. If he did not cease practicing, Reg would call the state chiropractic board and tell them the person was practicing chiropractic (mixing treatment or health practices with Spinology was chiropractic). He would not defend a Spinologist brought up on charges under these circumstances. By having this strict control, Reg knew that Spinology would not go the way of chiropractic, (i.e., mixing). What he did not foresee was that he would have to be a Spinology policeman, calling, writing, threatening and taking action against those who did not have the integrity to comply with the agreement that they had made in becoming a Spinologist, staying pure. This probably contributed to his decision to not continue Spinology. He did not want to spend his days trying to force people to practice something they should be practicing simply by having an understanding of the philosophy. When it came right down to it, Reg did not want to control people's lives, that is not his style, not when he had a philosophy, whether called straight chiropractic or Spinology, that would stand on its own merit.

Reg spent years at Columbia, Sherman and ADIO teaching chiropractic to college students, many of whom never had any intention of practicing straight chiropractic or who had drifted away from it for one reason or another shortly after leaving school. Spinology solved that problem but only by keeping control of the practitioner and counting on other Spinologists to turn in their friends who were practicing in a dishonest manner. Reggie did not count on the fact that many people came into Spinology with a secret agenda. They did not want to be "straight" Spinologists. Some had backgrounds in alternative therapies and much like the medical doctors who got into chiropractic at the turn of the century as well as throughout the history of the profession, they just wanted to add something else to their bag of tricks. That is not what Reg had in mind for Spinology. Reggie decided he did not want to police Spinology and force people to do something they should want to do. He decided to go back into chiropractic but not at the college level. He would present chiropractic through lectures, seminars, videos and audio tapes to those people who truly wanted straight chiropractic: those who would, of their own accord, choose it and who would seek him out to get it. Thus, the next phase of his life began.

CHAPTER 6

Getting Back into Chiropractic

1986-Present

While there were a number of reasons why Reg rejoined the straight chiropractic movement, perhaps the biggest was his deep, abiding love for chiropractic. Even though he has made major changes in its practice by his new vision of the philosophy and the fact that he did start Spinology, Reg has a loyalty to chiropractic. It gave him a perspective that has had a major impact upon his life. It enabled him to earn a very good living. He put it succinctly when he made the most extraordinarily generous of his many donations to Sherman in 1994, "Everything I am and have, I owe to chiropractic." Reggie had dozens of friends in chiropractic whom he was out of touch with during his years in Spinology. Rejoining the straight chiropractic movement also meant resuming many lifelong friendships.

It is important to note that it was no longer necessary for Reg to continue the effort and energy needed to sustain Spinology. It had served its purpose. Spinology had enabled Reg to present the non-therapeutic, non-health aspect of chiropractic care. Spinology's most important contribution may well have been to demonstrate that chiropractic could be practiced under another name in a non-therapeutic manner without any successful attacks from the medical or chiropractic community or any harassment from federal or state governmental agencies. Whatever happens to straight chiropractic in the future, the movement is assured that it can exist, as long as it does not purport to treat or cure disease or address health issues in a way that would necessitate governmental control. Spinology established forever a very important safety-valve for straight chiropractic which would assure, if not its name, at least the perpetuation of its philosophy and practice. The straight community owes a debt of gratitude to Reg for that service alone.

Despite the fact that Spinology had served its purpose, it was not fulfilling Reg's expectations for growth considering the amount of work he was putting into it. Spinology was growing but it was much more work than Reg had anticipated. Flying around the world, although glamorous to some, was time consuming, arduous work. Not that Reg has ever been afraid of work, but it was work that could not be delegated and there were simply not enough hours in the day. Fie had hoped to set up the tutoriums, put trustworthy people in charge and then just step away. Unfortunately, it was not that easy. It took constant care. Like the chiropractic profession, many in Spinology were prone to slipping and Reg was the only person who could really check the slipping. It became clear that moving straight chiropractic, which was already established, into his model of non-therapeutic care, would be a much more effective use of his time and energy.

Reggie needed straight chiropractic. His love was still with chiropractic, its historical roots and what it had given to him and had meant to his life. Spinology was straight chiropractic, although perhaps not straight chiropractic as practiced by most of the profession. It was definitely not chiropractic as defined by most state laws and was not the chiropractic that most practitioners understood. It was Reggie's vision of what straight chiropractic should be regardless of the name given to it.

It so happened at that time that the straight chiropractic movement was also in desperate need of help. The schools were struggling financially and it was no secret that Pennsylvania College and Southern California had some serious problems maintaining their straight philosophy. No one had even remotely replaced Reggie in his leadership position in the straight chiropractic community and certainly no one stepped forward as an articulate spokesperson for the profession. But more importantly, there was no one who could clearly and without compromise, present the vision of straight chiropractic who was not already totally occupied. The profession needed a traveling ambassador, spokesperson and conscience who could present chiropractic to students and chiropractors and bring those who had drifted, back to center. Sherman was having its problems, enrollment was down. Even the short-lived recognition of SCASA as an accrediting agency could not seem to boost enrollments or bring in the needed donations.

Reg knew that straight chiropractic could make it. The only things it lacked were numbers, a sense of purpose or mission and support for its institutions. He, more than anyone, had given those things for twenty-five years and had motivated others toward them. So Reg decided to get back into the straight chiropractic movement. It was done without any fanfare or formal announcements, he just began to speak to chiropractic groups. Wes Trout's Living Principles program was the first to publicly advertise Reg on the program, for which Wes received a great deal of criticism.

After that, Reggie was slowly invited to speak at other programs and his message was as true and inspiring as ever. Reg also took it upon himself to go to chiropractic colleges and speak to students. Wherever he went, he would promote Sherman and encourage chiropractors to donate to it and to send their prospective students there. Sherman people were somewhat perplexed. Why was Reggie on his own, often at his own expense, promoting Sherman College? The answer was simple; he did it because of his love for what the school represented. As matters grew increasingly bleak for Sherman and the straight movement, Reg stepped up his efforts. He stopped speaking about Spinology and began doing more and more chiropractic seminars. He was now fully back in the straight chiropractic movement, although he knew it would be awhile before those within the movement fully accepted him. Some chiropractors hold grudges for a long time and others are wary of chiropractors' motives in general. After a few years, Reg proved that his motivation was only to promote straight chiropractic. He continually gave and asked for nothing in return, often traveling to speak to groups at his own expense. He made no effort to get into positions of leadership, although the opportunities were there. He wanted no formal position in straight chiropractic, just to give of his knowledge. He began to get more and more speaking opportunities. Gary Dunn and Terry Rondberg started the Fountainhead Seminars, the first one taking place in Arizona. Reg was a key figure in the success of the program. When Palmer College threatened the program with legal action, claiming they owned the rights to the word "Fountainhead," the name was changed to ADIO Seminars. The program continued under that new name for a few years during which Reggie was often highlighted as a guest speaker.

Reggie also wanted a home, it is difficult for many to understand why someone would cut so many ties and bum so many bridges just to take a strong position like Reg has taken. Many chiropractors refuse to do it. There are hundreds of straight chiropractors who have never joined Reggie in the objective straight chiropractic movement because they could not stand to alienate themselves from Palmer, Life, Cleveland or another school to which they felt loyalty. Reggie, on the other hand, by taking his strong stand, became persona non-grata at many of those places, including his own alma mater.

Sherman became "home" for Reggie. Both the Living Principles and ADIO Seminars are no longer taking place and Reg has limited his speaking engagements almost entirely to those he sets up himself, with the exception of Sherman Lyceum and the New Beginnings program begun by Dr. Jim Dubell of Long Branch, New Jersey. Lyceum is the highlight of Reg's year. It is an opportunity for him to speak philosophically, to motivate chiropractors to greater support of the college and, most importantly, to rub shoulders with the largest group of chiropractors who think the way he does, because of his influence in many cases. Reg's association with Sherman since his return to the straight movement has evolved into a close, if unofficial, position. He is a goodwill ambassador for the school wherever he goes. He truly believes that Sherman College has and will continue to be the hub of the straight chiropractic community. Reg refuses to be critical of the recent changes that Sherman has made in the curriculum and in the Health Center to satisfy the CCE. He believes whatever they teach, as long as they maintain that those procedures are not part of the practice of straight chiropractic, that they are straight, and doing those things is only part of playing the game. Reg says it is no more of a compromise than teaching pathology and microbiology. Others in the straight community have been critical of Sherman, claiming it is doing exactly what the ICA schools did twenty years ago. The difference, as Reg sees it, is that those schools try to justify doing diagnostic procedures and incorporating diagnosis into the practice of chiropractic. While Sherman is now doing many of those same procedures, it does not try to rationalize them as part of the practice of chiropractic. Reg believes that they will continue to maintain that position, although it will become more and more difficult every year.

He also refuses to be critical of Sherman's intention to limit

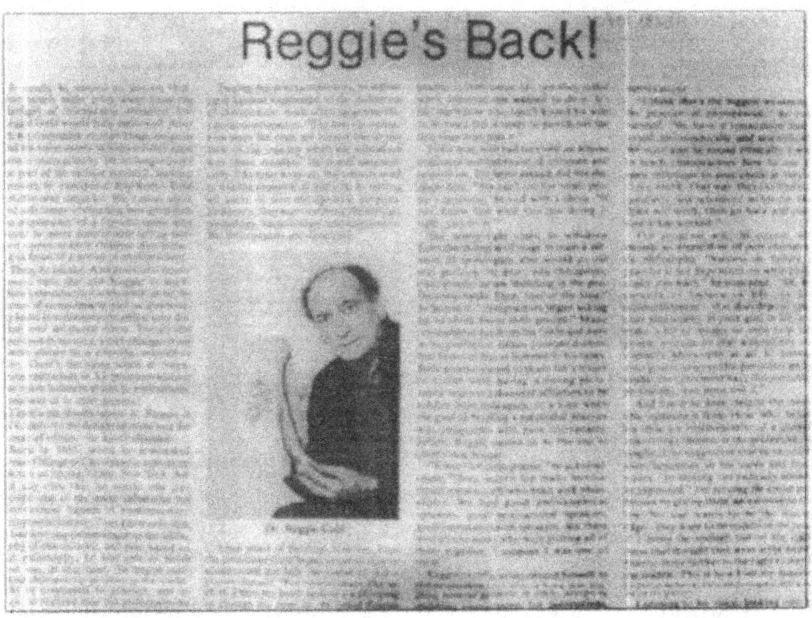

Reggie's Back!

The Chiropractic Journal, February 1988

class sizes as some in the straight chiropractic community are. The problem is that people misunderstand what they mean by "limit." To limit may imply that they could take more but choose not to. The fact is Sherman would take as many students as it possibly could (and maybe then some), at which point the tide of popularity would bring forth, naturally, new schools. Reg feels that when Sherman's enrollment nears the school's capacity, somewhere a new straight chiropractic college will emerge to fill the need. Already there is a straight chiropractic college in New Zealand, where one-fourth of the country's chiropractors are Sherman graduates. It is filling the need in that country. While some might disagree with Reggie and contend that we urgently need more straight schools right now to create the need for students, he maintains that when Sherman is filled, another school will emerge. The history of the straight chiropractic movement strongly favors Reggie's argument. Much of the problem with the straight schools in the past was a lack of a strong support base. There simply were not enough straight chiropractors to support Sherman, ADIO/Penn Straight, Southern California and SCASA. Reg maintains that if we can build a strong support base over the next few years, a new emerging straight school would only be in a better financial position to succeed. That is Reggie's desire and he is working on three fronts to see that come to fruition. First, he continues to support Sherman College financially in the area of recruitment and by lending his presence to its annual Lyceum. Secondly, Reg conducts his seminars around the country, almost every weekend, giving interested chiropractors a better understanding of the straight philosophy as well as the tools to practice it successfully. Thirdly, Reg is constantly speaking at chiropractic colleges (on or off campus) explaining what objective straight chiropractic is. It is amazing how positive many of the students at even the strong mixing schools are to his message. Many of these students come to chiropractic college not fully understanding what chiropractic is but knowing, for one reason or another, that they do not want to practice medicine. When they begin their education, they quickly learn that the school is trying to move chiropractic into the practice of medicine, either with or without the use of drugs. When they hear Reggie's message they often say "that makes complete sense." This occurs despite the fact that at many of these colleges the straight chiropractic approach is ridiculed and students are discouraged from hearing Reggie Gold.

In truth, Reggie came back to straight chiropractic from Spinology for one reason, the same reason that motivates him today, the perpetuation of the straight chiropractic principle. He began Spinology when he believed that opposition would overwhelm the schools and squelch the propagation of the philosophy. When it looked as if Sherman would make it, he came back. He was looking and continues to look for the best vehicle, the most effective means of perpetuating straight chiropractic. He has no qualms about starting another profession, he did that with Spinology. He has no reservations about using chiropractic and Sherman to meet that objective. It is not as if he alone shares that idea. Thom Gelardi himself has told Reg that Sherman's importance is only as a means to perpetuate straight chiropractic. Prior to going to Sherman in 1972, Reggie had been planning to start a post-graduate school and he maintains that the idea is still not beyond doing. He could see himself starting a six-month program in which graduates of non-straight schools could learn philosophy, patient education tools, communication skills and technique that they are obviously not getting in chiropractic school today. Reg feels that the current tremendous interest in low-force, non-force and non-contact techniques like DNFT, Activator, and Network is due largely to the fact that many chiropractors today are scared to death to put their hands on the patient. They have been so frightened by college faculty, malpractice insurance companies and risk management people into thinking that they are going to cause strokes, herniate disks and tear vertebral arteries that they have no confidence in their technique. Of course, the fact that so little time and emphasis is placed on technique in many chiropractic colleges may make legitimate their feeling of inadequacy. Reg thinks a post-graduate school would fill that void and, more importantly, would teach the deductive approach to chiropractic. Reggie has been and is still willing to do whatever it takes to further the philosophy and the practice of objective straight chiropractic.

Reg is optimistic that straight chiropractic may be finally turning the comer. He believes that the movement is picking up momentum and that in four or five years there will be enough straight chiropractors to support another straight school. One of the important aspects of the future of straight chiropractic is the change in the CCE. No longer is it being run by political people who follow the ACA thinking. Educators who apparently have no political ax to grind are now in control. Their desire is only to make sure that the institutions follow the highest educational standards possible. Of course, that has always been the desire of the straight chiropractic community. The only difference has been whether those standards should be chiropractic or medical. The CCE's leaders, despite being educators, still have a medical mindset. Reggie believes, as does Sherman, that these educators can "be convinced of the superiority of the objective straight approach or at least be tolerant of the non-diagnostic approach that forms the basis for its practice. As straight chiropractic grows, new schools can and will emerge to fill the need. Meanwhile, Sherman College can accommodate the referrals from the present straight chiropractic community.

Reggie and Sid Williams share the idea of filling the world with chiropractors but that is where their agreement ends. Sid has a traditional approach to chiropractic that also incorporates the need for diagnosis (which, for the record, is not part of the traditional approach to chiropractic). The size of Life College reflects Sid's passion. Reggie, on the other hand, sees the value of more schools with smaller classes allowing for individual attention, particularly in the area of technique. This is the goal of Sherman College. The ability to share the mission, the philosophy and the love of chiropractic is best served in a smaller, more closely knit environment, as Sherman College is gearing toward, rather than in extremely large classes. This is a departure for many in the straight chiropractic community who have grown up with the idea of volume practices, large schools and lots of chiropractors. Of course, this vision of Reg's depends upon the straight community having the people, the resources and the dedication to start new schools and enough straight chiropractors referring students to fill these. At the present time, it does not appear that the straight chiropractic community has any of them. So a new straight chiropractic college is still at least a few years away. Meanwhile, Reg works toward filling the classes at Sherman and converting chiropractors and students at non-straight schools to the objective straight approach. He does this by presenting straight chiropractic to the world. Reg's presentation has begun to focus more on practical issues, that is, "how to do it," rather than "why to do it." This is partly because he does not have to "convert" as many people as before with the fact that the philosophy just makes sense. Many of them are coming over on their own because of the frustrations and problems of a dying insurance practice, but they lack the tools to be successful as straight chiropractors. When he speaks to students at non-straight schools, Reg has to show them there is another way to practice, one that is in no way medical and yet rewarding in every way. So his presentation focuses almost entirely on the practical aspects. Of course, any presentation he does is liberally sprinkled with the chiropractic philosophy. Unfortunately, established chiropractors do not have the privilege of being exposed to Reggie unless they go to Sherman Lyceum or one of his seminars.

A number of chiropractors go to his seminars, some for licensure credits or to pick up a few ideas. A few end up walking away with an entirely new approach to chiropractic that changes their lives forever. One such case occurred recently in a seminar Reg did in Seattle. The chiropractor just needed his credits for Washington state. The Thursday after the weekend he called Reggie and said that he had completely changed his practice and had already signed up seven families on the family plan that Reg taught the previous weekend. Upon hearing Reggie, he realized that he was not really happy with his patch-up care practice and wanted a health-oriented family maintenance practice, the type Reggie was promoting.

There is no doubt Reggie changes lives with his message. He has been doing it from Spring Valley to the far comers of the earth.

But... perhaps if we can peel away some of the layers we can see the visionary in him, the teacher in him, and even the man himself - that small part of his personality that while linked to chiropractic is uniquely the private person. For as much as he is a public figure, there is much that is private about Reggie Gold.

Who is this Reggie Gold, and what makes him so powerful a force that he can change a chiropractor's practice and life in a week-end?

CHAPTER 7

Visionary/Teacher

Visionary

One with great dreams or projects.

Based on this definition alone, Reg is surely a visionary. He has had the ability to see in chiropractic what no one else has been able to see. He first gave us the vision of chiropractic to stay well. In the early sixties, this was a departure from the "chiropractic gets sick people well" that most of the profession practiced. That same decade he emphasized family maintenance care and by 1970 he had developed the non-therapeutic approach of chiropractic. Spinology solidified the idea that chiropractic care enhances potential in all areas of life. The chiropractic profession has had very few visionaries in its history. D.D. was, of course the first, he imagined the whole idea. B.J. was the greatest, but his focus was primarily on the practical ways to disseminate chiropractic. In recent times, there have been very few visionaries. Joe Flesia, Guy Riekeman and Thom Gelardi, Thom's vision primarily in the area of chiropractic education. Imagine the excitement at Sherman College in those days with the four of them there, Reggie, Joe, Guy and Thom! Perhaps the students were not really aware of the great minds they were tapping every day. Thom's vision continued in the area of education. His strong leadership skills were necessary to maintain the college through the difficult times that made up the first twenty-five years of its history. Joe and Guy ("Easy" as he was known in those days) had a vision in the Renaissance International program. They too were great thinkers. Joe has now settled into the Vertebral Subluxation Complex, its scientific underpinnings and trying to relate chiropractic to the scientific community. Guy, on the other hand, has moved into the area of practice management and self-improvement. While not strictly straight chiropractic, it is apparently something that many chiropractors need.

Reg could have easily stayed where he was at any point and been successful in practicing and promoting that particular model of chiropractic, but he is never satisfied. He is constantly trying to move on to new territories in the philosophy. He maintains that he is only trying to make it simpler, more easily understood by any intelligent lay person or chiropractor. While I'm sure that is true, I believe it is also because he wants to continually strike out into new and uncharted territories, simply because they are there to be explored. His life is one of trying things that supposedly cannot or have not been done. Whether it was joining an elite British regiment as a young Jew , smuggling guns to Israel, or seeing two thousand patients a week, he wants to do something no one else has done, thinks to do or can do. He is an explorer in the mold of a Lewis or Clark. Sure they were ostensibly trying to find a passage to the Pacific, but the challenge to them was to enter unknown territory, to blaze a path for others to follow. That is essentially what Reggie has been doing. Only instead of traveling through valleys and over mountains and rivers, he is traversing a philosophy, constantly trying to push further than anyone else has. Even his desire to simplify the chiropractic philosophy is a desire to do what no one has done, raise the percentage of people who understand chiropractic and subsequently, avail themselves of chiropractic care. While anxious to reach more people, Reggie remains realistic in his vision. It has been said that you can only walk half-way into the woods, then you are walking out. Many so-called "visionaries" in our profession have "blazed trails" past the center and are moving out of chiropractic or have moved out completely. Bill Bahan, one of the famous Bahan brothers from Derry, New Hampshire who made famous the "G.P.C. fee system," was one such visionary. He left chiropractic and began a religious concept called Ontology and taught it until his death. Reggie, however, is able to find the best trail to the center and only the center, no further. That has been his goal and each time he blazes a new trail, it is better than the last. He keeps trying to find the quickest and simplest route for all of humanity to the center of the chiropractic philosophy and no further. The more he simplifies and makes logical the message, the more thinking people will accept it. He is not divorced from reality, thinking that every person in the world will accept the idea of regular, lifetime care. But he is also not content to believe that chiropractic cannot reach more people than it now is or more people than anyone in the profession has ever dreamed.

There are two particular events that significantly encouraged the development of Reg, the visionary. The first, and perhaps the most important, was a comment made to him by a student attending one of his talks on the West Coast a number of years ago. Reg was talking about the mixers changing chiropractic to something other than what B.J. was doing. After his talk, the student came up to him and asked if he was not also changing chiropractic with the new philosophy that he was teaching.

It suddenly occurred to him that he was changing chiropractic and that maybe there really was nothing wrong with changing chiropractic. A philosophy should change and develop. B.J. had obviously changed it from D.D.'s cure for deafness and we can change it too, as long as the change is based upon the foundational principles of the Palmers (i.e., innate intelligence and vertebral subluxation). Also, it should be a change that is logical and one that does not impinge upon another healing art. Actually anyone is free to change chiropractic any way they want and for any reason but these three reasons seem to be the most honest and sensible. The Palmers do have some right to their discovery. Logic should always be a motivating force for change. There is no reason for chiropractic to become more like medicine if we already have medicine. So the change has to move us away from medicine.

Reg was going into unexplored territory with his philosophy but he was not unprepared. B.J. had given Reg the compass, so to speak. An explorer may enter into uncharted territory and blaze a trail for others to follow, but he has to have a goal in mind, a destination. He needs a compass to make sure he has not lost his bearing. Reggie has taken us to new areas in the chiropractic philosophy, but he has done it with B.J.'s compass. The compass is our major premise, the philosophy of innate intelligence, the idea of correcting vertebral subluxations, and the fact that we address DIS-EASE rather than disease. While Reggie has taken chiropractic far beyond where B.J. left it, into new territory, he has strongly relied upon that compass and has never disregarded it. That is the difference between the changes he has made and those that others have made. Even those that claim to practice the chiropractic of B.J. are into disease and its cause rather than DIS-EASE and its cause. For B.J. it was always DIS-EASE. Chiropractic has had to move, to change, Every profession changes. Baseball has changed in the past seventy-five years. Warfare has changed, medicine has changed, science has changed and even business practices have changed. Everything based on science and art must change. The question is, should chiropractic change by going into new areas still based upon the foundation of the chiropractic philosophy or by going back to the "safety" of the "civilized," accepted regions? The early settlers of this country entered new, uncharted territory. When they stepped on the shores of this country, it was an unknown area, but they ventured inland and took chances because they believed something better lay ahead. They knew what they had left in Europe and whatever lay ahead, had to be better than the poverty, oppression, overcrowding and disease that they had left behind. As Reggie ventured into a new area of the chiropractic philosophy and the practice of straight chiropractic, he knew it had to be better than the overcrowded field of therapeutic care. It had to be better than the oppression of medicine as a result of trying to compete with it for the disease treatment model. And it had to be better than waiting for people to get sick to make them better. That didn't mean it would be easy. There would be obstacles and there still are. There would be problems, some of Reggie's fellow trailblazers would even fall by the wayside. But Reg was able to foresee something better for chiropractic. Contrast the squalor of a European ghetto with the lush green of the Shenendoah Valley and you can appreciate what our early settlers must have seen in this country and what, by analogy, Reggie must see for the chiropractic profession. That is the mark of a visionary and sadly, a view all too few of us have.

The second event that freed Reggie to really open up his vision was Spinology. As mentioned earlier, when he left straight chiropractic, he was free of the "health field" and he could "broaden the scope" of his philosophy. Those that see chiropractic as a treatment for back problems have a limited vision. Those that see it as a treatment for disease and its cause have a broader but still limited vision. Those that see it as part of caring for health within the health field have a still broader yet still limited vision. It is true that if you define health as physical, mental and social well-being then it more closely resembles the vision that Reg has. Joe and Guy began doing this in the seventies. But it is also a sad fact that the American public still thinks of a health profession as one that deals with diseases, sickness and symptoms. When Reg went into Spinology, he was forced to totally abandon the health field and emphasize that Spinology had nothing to do with health. His position, though, was that it had *something* to do with *everything* else. That "everything else" was probably the broadest vision that could possibly be had. He could not have the freedom to do that under the banner of chiropractic, at least he did not feel he could. With chiropractic, he still had the old traditions that many chiropractors, even straight chiropractors, hang onto like being anti-medicine and getting sick people well. In Spinology, he was forced to abandon those traditions as well as every pretense of being chiropractic. The freedom he had to roam free in his vision and in his philosophical thinking could not have occurred otherwise. When he came back to chiropractic, he was able to bring that back with him. He would never be the same having had the vision of what chiropractic could be, if it was unfettered like Spinology. I'm sure those that explored the wilderness of this country hundreds of years ago were never the same when they returned to civilization. Imagine, three hundred years ago, trying to explain to someone who lived all their life in a crowded London slum that there were wide open spaces for as far as you could see. That there were green mountains and lakes and streams and all kinds of wildlife and that you could walk for two weeks and not reach the mountains that lay in the distance. Television and travel magazines have made it hard for us to relate to someone simply explaining their vision of far off places, but in the 17th and 18th century, it was quite different. Many of these explorers were so graphic and convincing in their description of the new world that they persuaded hundreds, even thousands, of others to go back with them to explore and eventually settle in this unknown, uncharted land. I believe that is Reggie's role. He has seen what chiropractic can be, not necessarily what it can do, but what it can be. Now he wants to share that vision with every other chiropractor and convince them to travel with him to a better life in chiropractic. That is the visionary in Reg Gold. He sums it up best himself. "Without being a visionary, I wouldn't be anything. It is what gives me something to talk about. You have to see what doesn't exist. Any idiot can see what's there, to describe what's there, so what. To be able to see what is not yet there and be able to shape it in your mind so clearly that you can see it and share it with other people, a visionary yes, but that is also what makes me a teacher."

Teacher

Vision is pretty much worthless unless you can share it.

Reg Gold

When people think of Reggie Gold, most think of his ability to share chiropractic. Few realize that he has actually put many of these great philosophical concepts together himself. This is not only due to the fact that Reg rarely engages in self-proclamation but also, and mostly due to the fact that his ability to clearly and simply explain those concepts is so impressive. Reg began as a teacher at Columbia in the early sixties and to this day still considers himself above all, a teacher. He gave up practice to teach at Sherman because he felt he had a special talent for teaching. Many people can become good chiropractors but only a few have the ability to teach. In addition to Columbia and Sherman, he also taught at ADIO and the Spinology Tutorium. In the last few years, Reg's teaching has taken on a new direction. While there are only a few who have a special talent for teaching, there are even fewer who have the ability to teach people who believe they already have a knowledge of the subject taught. That is by far the most difficult challenge in teaching. Reggie has a unique ability to cut through people's pseudo-understanding and present them with the truth of the matter. He can enable people to say, "That makes perfect sense. Why didn't I think of that before?" and "How could

I have been so wrong all this time?" He allows people to see the truth for themselves. Many teachers draw pictures for people sitting with their eyes closed in order to get them to understand. These people rarely have much success. Reg has the ability to get people to open their eyes, to take a glimpse at his picture. Some of them do not like what they see because it conflicts with their current understanding or their financial or status desires. But many are changed, often for the rest of their lives. That ability makes Reggie Gold a teacher among teachers. With this talent, he can go where other chiropractic teachers cannot go. He can open the eyes of disenchanted mixers and students from strong mixing schools. Many times, he has even changed those who saw no need to change. Mixer chiropractors and chiropractic students who are perfectly happy in their practices have come to hear Reg speak, perhaps out of curiosity. Reg has turned even some of *them* around, making them realize that although their lives and practice seem successful, they really lack clear direction, true purpose and the ability to make an impact upon every person with whom they come in contact. It is easy to change the mixer who is dissatisfied with practice and life or who is failing in practice. It is difficult to reach the ones who are successful by most people's standards and who are even remotely happy in practice. Reg has that ability. Apparently there is a place in the heart of every person that can be touched by idealism, that responds to a logical presentation and that is impacted by a simple, clear message. Reg has the ability to touch that place.

Some have suggested that Reggie should be teaching at a chiropractic college exposing seventy-five or a hundred students to a daily regimen of chiropractic philosophy in a deductive manner. He could be doing that if he so chose. But he has refused to do it. "There is no need for me to do that. There are a lot of my former students teaching philosophy in chiropractic colleges." Perhaps when the schedule that he now keeps, doing his seminars and speaking On and off campus at chiropractic colleges, becomes too exhausting, he will go back to private practice and teach at a chiropractic college. (He still believes that chiropractic college faculty should first be successful practitioners.) Meanwhile, he has plenty of energy to keep up the pace of traveling almost fifty-two weeks a year. What he is doing now is awakening or opening the eyes of ten times as many students as he would in the classroom. Touching the lives of seventy-five students over and over for thirteen weeks would be great but stirring a desire to investigate more and more about straight chiropractic in thousands of students at Canadian Memorial, Life, LACC, Logan and Western States is so much more. Reg can impassion people with wanting more out of the practice of chiropractic and out of their life, more than they ever realized, people who might otherwise never even know there was more to have. That ability would be limited in the classroom.

Another teaching skill that Reg possesses like no other chiropractor is the ability to bring straight chiropractors back to center. The nature of straight chiropractic lends itself to slipping. The philosophy is within finely defined lines and even the best of chiropractors slips from time to time. Often we do not have the ability to check that slipping because it is so slight that we don't even realize we have slipped. Eventually however, that slipping, if not checked will cause the chiropractor to lose his or her entire focus. What may start out as a small thing, such as allowing patients to share their symptoms without reminding them of your objective, ends up as adding modalities to treat their symptoms. That may be an extreme example but it has actually happened many times. Reggie can check people's slipping perhaps better than any chiropractor alive, mostly because he is totally centered on chiropractic. He does not water down his message even one little bit. He is also the master at checking others' slipping because of his ability to impassion people. Losing your passion predisposes you to slipping. Reg can ignite the flame of passion to change yourself, your practice, your community and the world. Lastly, his ability to check others' slipping is due partly to the fact that you always learn something new every time you listen to Reg. I have never heard him speak over the past thirty-two years that I did not come away with at least one new thought. It may not even have been that Reggie said anything different, but I was a different person every time I heard him so he was able to reach me at a different level. And so he does each time I hear him speak.

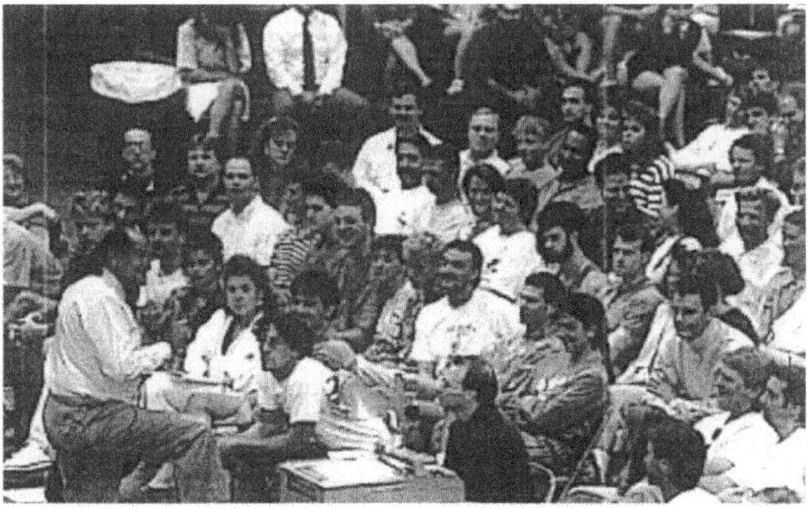

Reggie speaking to a group of Palmer students

It is sad that Sherman College Lyceum is made to be such a "Sherman event" and that many straight chiropractors from other schools do not feel totally comfortable there. It is the only place to hear Reggie Gold speak on a regular basis. It is true that he has many speaking engagements over the course of the year, but on any given occasion it might not be conveniently located, the chiropractor may not know about it or he may be unable to go. Most chiropractors who are successful and running busy practices will not take the time to attend one of his seminars, especially if they think it is for those who want to turn their practices around. Yet, I believe that every straight chiropractor should hear Reggie speak at least once a year. For as long as I can remember, Memorial Day weekend has been reserved for Spartanburg, South Carolina on Reggie's calendar. Part of the weakness of the straight chiropractic movement may well be that those within it do not get enough of Reggie to bring them back to center and unfortunately, there are few other people capable of doing it like him.

Reggie is one of, if not the most, creative thinkers in the chiropractic profession. It has been said that creativity is really the recalling of truth. Columbus was a creative person, taking three ships of about fifty feet in length on a voyage across uncharted waters to find a route to India, when much of the world thought that the earth was flat. For centuries prior to Columbus, however, many people knew the earth was a globe. The Vikings made the trip before Columbus and others probably did also. Columbus merely recalled and brought to light a truth that may have been known since the formation of the earth. Reggie's creativity has been in his ability to bring to light the truth of chiropractic. The chiropractic philosophy that Reggie espouses has always existed. It was present in the first adjustment by D.D. Palmer. It just took someone to draw it out of D.D.'s and B.J.'s ideas. Reggie has been able to do that. The other area where his creativity is demonstrated is in drawing analogies and ideas to explain chiropractic in more simple terms. In his quest to simplify and make logical the chiropractic philosophy, Reg has developed numerous analogies and metaphors to explain chiropractic. He has touched many, many more people in this way. In 1996,I published a book for lay people entitled *Enhance your Life Experience.* In that book is a short story - "Digging Up Holes." It draws the analogy between a hole in the ground being the absence of dirt in the same way that disease is merely an absence of health. To get rid of a hole you do not try to dig it up, you merely replace the dirt. Yet, the outside-in approach of health care is to get rid of disease rather then restore health, a state of harmonious function within the body. The idea for that short story came from a statement Reggie made as the banquet speaker at a Chiropractic Fellowship of

Pennsylvania annual convention back in the early seventies. It was a simple statement. I do not recall ever hearing it before or since, yet it stuck with me for over twenty years and precipitated the writing of that short story. Without doubt, any straight chiropractor who is speaking to patients, doing orientations or lay lectures, is using one or more of the analogies that Reggie has developed to more clearly explain the philosophy of straight chiropractic.

Of all Reggie's stories, analogies and metaphors, without doubt his most famous and most well-known is the "Valley of the Blind" talk. This talk was first given at a Palmer Homecoming in the early sixties. Interestingly, however, its message is just as powerful and just as relevant today as it was thirty-five years ago. The original story, *The Valley of the Blind,* written by H.G. Wells, is about an explorer who is hopelessly lost and accidentally stumbles into a remote village cut off for generations from the outside world where everyone is blind. They have no knowledge of the concept of eyesight and actually fear and mistrust the explorer. By the end of the story, the main character who believed he would be a hero to the village when first arriving is told he must give up his eyesight to be accepted into society.

Chiropractors were in the same place in the sixties and are still there in 1997. They are asked to give up, not their eyesight, but their vision. The vision of chiropractic is to correct vertebral subluxations to allow the innate intelligence of the body to be better expressed for as many people as possible. That includes sick people, healthy people, people at play, people at work, old, young and everyone else. Chiropractors are being asked to give this up and to take care of only people with bad backs so they can be paid by insurance companies or the government. Like the character in the story, chiropractors are not having their vision taken away, they are agreeing to give up their vision for acceptance. To Reg, acceptance at the price of giving up your principles, your philosophy and your vision is too costly. He has maintained this position and this message for the past quarter of a century, making the "Valley of the Blind " talk as important today as it was when it was first given.

Almost every straight chiropractor uses or has used something taken from Reggie Gold. His analogies, stories and explanations of chiropractic lend themselves to being copied. If imitation is the sincerest form of flattery, then Reggie is without doubt the most flattered chiropractor in the world. But it is the simplicity of his philosophy that everyone would love to appropriate. How does he make it so simple?

CHAPTER 8

The Philosophy

Reggie has done more to develop, to refine and to communicate chiropractic philosophy than any person in the history of the profession. That is not meant to belittle the work of B.J. Reg himself admits that he has only been able to define chiropractic because he has had the advantage of almost sixty years of B.J.'s groundwork. The Developer faced unique obstacles, situations and a very different environment and because of that he was able to develop chiropractic to the place it was in 1961. Any one who fails to understand history is unable to make effective changes in the future. Reg understood the historical development of chiropractic by B.J., and to some degree D.D., but he also had the insight to see that the world is different today and that chiropractic cannot camp at the grave side of its ancestors. We must keep moving forward and keep developing, but without compromising the objective.

One area that benefited Reg was the opportunity to teach in chiropractic college. There is nothing that makes your arguments stronger and more effective than refining them in the caldron of the classroom. There are always students who want to challenge the instructor. In a straight chiropractic school, there are always those who want to punch holes in the philosophy. Some because they don't accept it and others for a very legitimate reason. Before these students commit the rest of their lives to doing something, they want to make sure it is totally valid. The philosophy is the only thing that validates the practice of chiropractic. Reg was constantly refining his presentation, creating new analogies and ways to get it across more effectively. That is the real key to his presentation, his ability to simplify the message, to bring it down to the most easily understood and accepted concept possible.

Defining Chiropractic by its Objective

The idea of defining chiropractic by its objective did not come as a revelation to Reg. It evolved, but it was largely in place by the time he left practice and had gone to South Carolina. It probably came about in response to questions at his Saturday night sessions in Spring Valley. Many great questions were asked there and in response to those questions, new concepts and ideas were developed. There was one particular chiropractor's wife who was a nutritionist and who would constantly question Reg about the importance of nutrition and why straight chiropractors ignore nutrition in their practices. Those coming to the sessions were at various levels of understanding. In addition, as word spread of these meetings, more and more chiropractors would show up. They saw the new enthusiasm of their friends and/or the positive changes in their practices and wanted to find out what was going on in Spring Valley to cause these changes. Because of this, Reg was forced to continually go back to basics and to repeat the principles he had already taught. It also caused him to constantly try to simplify the message, to get it across as quickly as possible, so he could move on to newer ideas and to give those regular attendees a new way of hearing the same philosophy. In doing this and in response to the nutritionist, this idea of defining chiropractic by its objective came about.

This, of course, was a major breakthrough in chiropractic philosophy and a real departure from the traditional definition of chiropractic as composed by B.J. and taught in Stephenson's *Chiropractic Textbook.* At once it eliminated the mixing that was being done under the guise of "things natural" in B.J.'s definition. This became the response to the nutritionist and to anyone else who felt what they had to offer people in the way of health care was valuable and should be incorporated into the chiropractor's practice. Chiropractic did not pass judgment on the value of any other procedure. It just was not chiropractic and to mix it with chiropractic was, well, it was mixing. This objective, non-judgmental approach to chiropractic had a number of new ramifications. If all procedures, other than the correction of vertebral subluxations to allow the innate intelligence of the body to be expressed more fully, were not chiropractic, and if incorporating them into chiropractic practice was mixing, then chiropractors could not judge the value of these procedures. Admittedly, there are other things and procedures beside an adjustment that benefit the human organism, including exercise, nutrition and even medicine and surgery. However, if they are not chiropractic and we do not do them, then we are not in a position to judge their value, especially for any particular individual. This new objective approach has, in principle, removed the animosity between straights and mixers. In other words, being a mixer is no longer judged as being bad. It is just not straight chiropractic.

Sometime back, the president of the ICA suggested that we do away with the terms "straight" and "mixer." That is not necessary as long as there is no negative connotation to being one or the other. They are simply two different ways to practice. If people have truly listened to Reggie's message since this objective approach has become his standard, they have heard a non-judgmental approach. Granted, it has not been accepted and/or applied by all of the objective straight chiropractic community. Old prejudices are hard to break for some, but by and large, the objective straight chiropractor has accepted the right of the mixer to do his thing. Of course, this acceptance also necessitates the acceptance of medical procedures and not judging the practice of medicine, including drugs and surgery. Reggie no longer suggests that, for example, the practice of medicine is bad as he once did quite adamantly. The traditional straight and the conservative mixer, on the other hand, show no such tolerance to those of our profession who want to incorporate prescription drugs and minor surgery. If we are to do away with the term "mixer" as the ICA president suggested, how shall we classify those who want to prescribe? Similarly, the traditional straight and the conservative mixer are still very antagonistic toward the medical profession.

One can see that defining chiropractic by its objective has tremendous benefit. It clearly defines the profession better than it has ever been in the past. Defining chiropractic also allows for other approaches, so long as they do not pretend to be straight chiropractic. Lastly, it does not pass judgment on any medical or therapeutic procedure. It is one of the great breakthroughs of the chiropractic profession.

The Chemistry of Life

The lecture entitled "The Chemistry of Life" is to date Reggie's greatest contribution to a lay explanation of chiropractic. That is not to say that in the future he will not come up with a clearer explanation of chiropractic, but this talk definitely presents the essence of the objective straight chiropractic philosophy as we have come to know it. It is difficult to say how "The Chemistry of Life" talk developed. For Reg, it was not something that came to him in a brilliant moment of enlightenment. Perhaps B.J. was the only person who had "thot flashes." Reggie admits that most of his ideas have come slowly after evolving in his mind over a period of time. As a result, Reg does not often stand up and announce to his audience and the world that he has a new, brilliant idea. Usually his ideas are presented as an evolution or an extension of his past thinking and one who listens to him often would hardly realize that his thinking or presentation has changed. Many people think Reggie is saying the same thing he did twenty-five years ago because they have heard him speak a hundred times. However, if you were to compare a talk from 1971 with one from 1996, you would see a tremendous difference in his presentation and his message.

Because Reg builds idea upon idea, he has never received the credit he deserves as a seminal thinker in chiropractic. Yet to take an idea from someone like B.J. and to develop it into a more philosophically sound, more logically arguable concept in such a way as to make it more easily understood by either a lay person or a chiropractor takes just as much genius as to come up with the original thought. In some ways, it is even more difficult. As Reggie's thinking has slowly evolved, he has given more thought to his philosophy and ways to communicate it and to make sure it strikes a chord in the logical mind and conforms to our deductive philosophy. As a result, Reggie has presented very little in the way of chiropractic thought that has been controversial or has created divisions in the straight chiropractic community. It has often been said that Reggie is a controversial character. While that may be true, it is certainly not because his message is controversial. If you have a non-medical or non- therapeutic objective, you must come to a logical conclusion. That is because Reggie's argument is well thought out and well developed. B.J., on the other hand, was truly controversial. He came up with ideas that perhaps were not so well thought through. It was his "innate thot flash" idea that made him think that any idea he had was automatically right and was needed by the entire profession. History shows that two such ideas, the NCM and HIO, caused great rifts in the profession. While many chiropractors have not followed Reg's lead in chiropractic, it has never been because the idea did not make sense to them.

Reggie was talking about body chemistry as early as 1972. In a radio interview done that year for a PACE chapter in Springfield, Massachusetts, the radio personality, a man by the name of Don Edwards shared his own personal physical ailment, a skin condition. In challenging him to see a chiropractor, Reg said, "What's happening is that an imbalance in body chemistry causes the problem. If emotional pressure caused the condition, then everybody in your business would have the condition. First, there must be a gradual lessening of the efficiency of the body chemically, which is followed by a breakdown or weakening of the organs... But it will never be corrected until body chemistry is restored to balance... Health generally is regulated by chemicals, body chemistry, hormones in balance or out of balance. The manufacture of every hormone, every chemical in the body, is regulated by nerves..." As a side note, Edwards took

Reggie's challenge and saw the PACE chapter advisor. A few weeks later, he was back on the air testifying that his twenty-five year old skin problem, which he had been treating for six years with corticosteroids, had cleared up under chiropractic care.

The Chemistry of Life explanation developed more fully in Spinology. Reg wanted to give an explanation for the need for Spinology that was different from chiropractic. Like other ideas of Reg's, it evolved. Spinology dealt with human potential. That was what separated it from chiropractic. When Reg came back to chiropractic, he just took the explanation a little further. He went from explaining how human potential was dependent upon body chemistry to explaining how vertebral subluxations affect body chemistry, which affect human potential. It was an inevitable development because it was such a logical sequence. Reg was consciously trying to simplify chiropractic, as well as his explanation, as to why everyone should be adjusted regularly and he felt that keeping body chemistry normal was something that everyone could relate to. Thus, through this one explanation, both the shoe salesman and the Ph.D. in biochemistry could see the importance of regular chiropractic care.

In the Chemistry of Life talk, Reg avoids the use of the term innate intelligence and instead uses terms like "nature" and "the body." He believes that while an understanding of the innate intelligence is important in a person's long-term commitment to regular chiropractic care, it can be confusing on the initial orientation. He wants the patient to understand subluxation and why it is important to have subluxations corrected on a regular basis. He advocates a continuing education program for all patients in which the concept of innate intelligence and other important chiropractic concepts can be taught. There are six lectures in the series including deduction, the Major Premise and innate intelligence. He advocates an initial lecture that does not include the concept of innate intelligence because very few chiropractors can explain it without causing at least some confusion for the patient. Either they present it so that it interferes with the patient's religious concepts or they present it as a religious thing that offends the non-religious people. Reg says "It (innate intelligence) is just not necessary for people to understand why they are better off not subluxated." Reg's major emphasis is getting the children to grow up subluxation-free. He believes it is possible to explain this without having to get into innate intelligence.

One of the things that has concerned Reggie over the years is the fact that many patients espouse a "belief" in chiropractic. Granted some of this is due to the patient's inability to express their understanding and acceptance of the logic of chiropractic. However, some of it does border on a belief. Innate intelligence seems to precipitate this problem. Telling people things they already know and pointing out how subluxation interferes with those things does not necessitate any belief. Reg sometimes begins "The Chemistry of Life" talk using the analogy of a food processor and how you get your money's worth from it only after you begin to learn more about it and what it can do. He has also used a television as the analogy and how it may be used as a plant stand if you know nothing of how it works versus a 180 cable channel entertainment system with video games. These analogies are extremely vital in getting the patient to understand straight chiropractic. Twenty-five years ago, it was not necessary because the public knew little about chiropractic. But with so many people going to chiropractors for back problems and so much advertising of musculoskeletal conditions being "treated" by chiropractors, advertising that was illegal thirty years ago, it is now necessary to "re"educate people. The most difficult thing in education is to teach someone a concept that they mistakenly believe they already know. So to start the talk, Reg compliments the listener by implying they know about chiropractic. Then, he humbly suggests that he may have something to add to that knowledge so that they can receive more benefit from chiropractic care, just as they would get more benefit from the food processor or the television if they understood all the things that they could do.

Interestingly, Reg does not ignore the fact that most people go to a chiropractor for back problems. Too often, straight chiropractors start off by telling the new patient or the prospective patient that chiropractic is *not* for back problems. This can be confusing to the patient and may even be a turn off especially if every contact they have had with chiropractors or with chiropractic (advertising) has been related to back problems. So Reg starts by recognizing that his listeners may already know about chiropractic but then continues by saying he is going to explain something more. The talk also acknowledges that people go to chiropractors for organic problems (e.g., high blood pressure, low blood pressure, arthritis) but then explains that even this does not scratch the surface of what chiropractic can do for people. After explaining that chiropractic is more than a way to get well, he says, "What I want to tell you tonight is that chiropractic, properly used, has nothing to do with backaches and it has nothing to do with any of those disease conditions that I have mentioned."

In the first five minutes of the talk, Reg has explained that:

1. Chiropractic is more than the listener thinks it is.
2. People get well from various medical conditions under chiropractic care and going to a chiropractor will help you recover from those problems.
3. If you are using chiropractic care for that purpose alone, you are wasting 98% of its real value.

With that as an introduction, Reg then explains how understanding more about how the body works will help them to understand more about chiropractic. Chiropractic deals not just with the health potential of the body, but with every physical activity of the body. Chiropractic relates to every level of human performance because every level of human performance is controlled by body chemistry. Here is where Reg has introduced one of the newest and most important concepts in patient education. Previously, chiropractic had avoided talking about body chemistry. That was the field of medicine. Chiropractors affected the nervous system by adjusting, while medical doctors alter body chemistry by giving drugs. Chiropractic traditionally has avoided talking about changing the chemistry of the body because it was thought to be mechanistic. Here, for the first time to my knowledge, was someone attempting to bridge the gap between the chemistry-changing mechanistic model of medicine and the neural-normalizing vitalistic model of chiropractic. Reggie points out in this talk that medicine is not wrong for trying to change body chemistry in the treatment of disease. Chemical imbalance is often the cause of the problem. The fault of medicine lies in the way they are trying to go about it. They are educatedly trying to balance something that only the innate intelligence of the body can know for sure. Further, if normalizing body chemistry is effective in restoring health then maintaining normal body chemistry would seem to be an effective approach to maintaining not only health but normal body function in general. He explains how your body chemistry "determines how much energy you have in the course of a day, how well you sleep at night, your moods, your attitudes and how well you get along with other people." He continues with plenty of examples. One of Reggie's greatest abilities is to pick out simple, every day examples to which anyone and everyone can relate and can apply to a major point of philosophy in order to gain a totally new way of looking at life or health or an important universal truth. His ability to explain profound truth with simple everyday experiences and concepts to which everyone can relate is what makes his presentation so powerful.

"You cannot get up in the morning and run for the bus without first changing your body chemistry." The body pumps adrenaline into your bloodstream to enable you to increase performance. "When you change body chemistry, you change performance. It takes chemicals to fall asleep at night and if your body is not producing a sufficient quantity of those chemicals all the time you will have periodic insomnia. If you take a chemical into your body such as coffee, you can upset that chemical balance and have the same result. People take chemicals to go to sleep and then have a difficult time waking up because the body is not producing a sufficient quantity to overcome the disturbance to its chemistry."

Reg moves the listener from the body producing chemicals for performance to producing chemicals to keep you healthy. "There are hundreds of different carcinogens, cancer-producing drugs in the food you eat, the air you breathe and the water you drink. How then do you manage to survive? You survive by making the right chemicals." Because everyone knows good nutrition is important for good health, he then applies the chemical making process to gaining nutrition from the food that we eat. Most lay people think that the food they eat determines their nutrition. While the food is important, it is the chemicals that our body produces to extract the nutrients from the food we eat that determines whether they have nutritional value to us. Most lay people are familiar with the term "enzymes" but many do not realize that the body produces enzymes to break down food for nutritional purposes. Reg says, "You may think you are what you eat. That's not true. You are what your body is able to extract from what you eat." If your body chemistry is not working as it should, all the good food in the world will not benefit you.

Reg continues to make the point that you need chemicals for everything. He uses examples of alcohol and the commonly used dental anesthetic, nitrous oxide, to explain that body chemistry can make you laugh, alter your moods or affect your coordination and your reaction time. In the case of alcohol, your judgment may be affected, you may even be unable to see straight or think straight. Interestingly, changes in body chemistry affect every body differently. Under the influence of alcohol some people can become friendly and jovial, others become angry and belligerent.

Reggie uses a classic and proven method of teaching, he attaches the thing to be learned (the yet unknown) to something familiar (known), making the unknown seem familiar and easier to recall. An example that he has made famous is hay fever. While most people believe that ragweed pollen causes hay fever, it is really due to an imbalance in body chemistry. When there is pollen in the air, the body responds by creating histamine. If the body produces too much histamine, the symptoms of hay fever occur. From this example comes the classic quote, "If ragweed pollen caused hay fever, we would all have hay fever." I do not remember when I personally first heard that statement, but it is so simple and profound that you have to wonder how many lives would change if every person could hear that one statement. He goes on to say that when body chemistry is out of balance, the entire body works improperly and that drugs, even those that are given to treat a condition like hay fever, upset the body's chemical balance and affect all the functions controlled by body chemistry. The logical conclusion is that if you are taking drugs, legal or illicit, your body will suffer the adverse effects of an upset chemistry.

He also uses the example of the menstrual cycle, which many people can identify with, at least to some degree. Reg's point is that the cycle corresponds with changes in female chemistry. Those changes in turn cause physical changes such as water retention, complexion problems and the emotional extremes often associated with "PMS." Just as low blood sugar can make people irritable because of an empty stomach (i.e., chemical change), chemical changes due to changing female hormones can alter mood. Diseases like Parkinson's and Alzheimer's are also related to chemistry, specifically the lack of a particular chemical in the brain. Everyone has heard of these diseases and so can easily bring to mind the direct results of a lack of proper chemistry. These are simply problems with body chemistry, regardless of the name placed upon them. Reg takes the medical profession's own concepts of disease and reduces them to a lack of balance in the body's chemistry. He literally demonstrates the junction where the DIS-EASE of chiropractic, (the lack of ease in the body), and the disease of medicine meet. Medicine cannot accept the DIS-EASE concept as we present it (incoordination in the nervous system), but they can surely accept the idea of a lack of balance in the body's chemistry.

Reg proceeds to make the natural transition from how chemicals outside the body can affect performance to how chemicals produced within the body can affect performance, especially if they are not being produced properly. He uses hyperthyroidism and hypothyroidism as examples. His emphasis is not so much on the disease as it is its effect upon performance, (i.e., not having enough energy to perform one's job, in the case of hypothyroidism). Reg then makes a smooth transition from chemical imbalance interfering with performance to the cause of illness within the body. "Now there are 70,000 billion cells in your body and every one of them is a little chemical factory." The chemicals necessary to adapt the body to the environment and keep your body's resistance high are made within the body. If the chemistry gets out of balance, you lose the ability to fight off bacteria and viruses. This is why at certain times your resistance is very high while at other times your resistance is low, "Run down means out of balance."

By this time, Reg is well into his talk and it is time to introduce chiropractic. "How does body chemistry relate to chiropractic? For you to make the right chemicals, they have to be controlled by a master control system. That system is the nervous system. How do the glands and organs that produce the chemicals know that a particular chemical is needed in a distant part of the body? All parts of the body are constantly feeding information concerning their status and their needs to the brain and the brain, in turn, is sending out messages to the chemical factories to respond to the body's needs." He then goes on to explain the function of the brain and spinal cord and their importance to the running of the body. He uses the creation of the body from two little half-cells, explaining that the first organ to appear is what will be the brain and spinal cord, the communication system of the body. He notes that only after the nerves have developed, do the organs and glands that will produce the chemicals of the body begin to develop. The body does not develop parts until there is a master control system for them. Since these organs (the brain and spinal cord) are that important and are not replaceable, chiropractors suggest that you take good care of them.

The electrical energy generated by the brain determines whether you are alive or not. It is so important that nature has protected it with bone, the skull and the vertebral column. If these bones are where they belong, the nervous system functions as it should, the messages reach the glands and organs and the body chemistry is as it should be. You can then adapt to every stimulus in the environment. Reg notes, "That doesn't mean you are going to be as good as the next guy but you are as good as you can be."

Subluxation interferes with the body's perfect coordination and consequently causes an imbalance in the body's chemistry. Subtle changes in chemistry result in our inability to adjust to the environment as quickly as we should. For example, we may be unable to get the maximum benefit from the food we eat. When your nervous system is functioning properly, your body chemistry is under control and you are better off. Reg then explains how subluxations occur, using the same examples that he has been using for years. Most chiropractors use every day adult activities to explain to adults how they can become subluxated. But Reg's explains how adults have probably been subluxated since childhood! The point he makes is that the effects may take years, but an uncorrected subluxation will "mess up your entire life." Your ability to work, concentration, digestion and your capacity for life in general are all affected by vertebral subluxation. Reg emphasizes that while we have not proved that subluxation causes anything, it simply is not necessary to prove it. Subluxation interferes with every function and activity of your life to some degree and that itself is enough to necessitate that all subluxations be corrected. This leads to two important points. First, the importance of chiropractic care for children. By explaining how subluxations occur in childhood, Reg has already set the stage for the importance of having children adjusted on a regular basis. Second, since subluxations do not hurt, you cannot know that you have them, and hence, the importance of regular chiropractic care for life. Reg confides, "I go to a chiropractor to have my spine checked at least once a week." He emphasizes, not sickness and disease, but the lessening of all human potential. Subluxation effects every aspect of life, consequently, you and your entire family need regular, lifetime chiropractic maintenance care.

Reg also briefly talks about the patient's responsibility to tell others about the need for chiropractic. He uses an example from his own practice of a man who had been bringing his asthmatic son to the office for care for only a short time when he met a neighbor of his who had been under care for nine years. He asked his neighbor why he had never suggested he bring his son into the office, despite knowing the boy had been rushed to the hospital on more than one occasion due to asthmatic attacks. You owe it to your friends and neighbors to tell them about chiropractic. He summarizes with his famous letter "N" explanation.

1. Chiropractic deals with human performance.
2. Every level of human performance is controlled by body chemistry.
3. Body chemistry is controlled by the glands whose job it is to make chemicals.
4. All the glands are controlled by the nerve system.
5. The nerve system is protected by the bones of the spine.

A subluxation occurs.

1. A vertebral subluxation is a bone over which the body has lost some of its control.
2. The position of the bone irritates the nerves.
3. Irritated nerves disrupt gland function.
4. Improper gland function disrupts body chemistry.
5. Disrupted body chemistry decreases performance levels.

A chiropractic adjustment is given.

1. A chiropractic adjustment restores proper bony position.
2. Proper position of the bone removes nerve irritation.
3. Restored nerve control allows for normal gland function.
4. Proper gland production balances body chemistry.
5. Proper/balanced body chemistry increases performance.

At this point in the talk, Reggie presents what is the hallmark of his presentation and what may very well be the most important contribution to chiropractic since D.D.'s discovery in 1895. An adjustment may not make your symptoms go away but it is not meant to. An adjustment opens up the life channels of your body and improves your overall life and it does that every time in every body. Of course, the important point is that people should want that for themselves with or without medical problems and regardless of whether those medical problems improve, stay the same or get worse under chiropractic care. In other words, chiropractic is not about your diseases or lack of diseases, it is about your life.

Here he makes a further argument for regular care. The damage done to the body's overall ability to be healthy is cumulative. If you get adjusted the day after you are subluxated that is not too bad, a month later, that is not too good, thirty years later some of the damage may be permanent. For the maximum benefits of chiropractic care, begin as early in life as you possibly can and do it for a lifetime.

Reggie's lasting contribution to the chiropractic profession will be the hundreds, possibly thousands of chiropractors whose lives and practices have been changed by his message, including his presentation of the "Chemistry of Life." It will also be the millions of people's lives that will be affected by the adjustments given by those chiropractors. My books, which could not have been written without the knowledge passed on to me by Reg, are also a tangible contribution by Reg, for at least as long as the chiropractic profession sees value in them. With something that evolves as the chiropractic philosophy has, it is questionable as to how long any presentation will have value other than as an historical document. Reg himself acknowledges this in a advertisement for Chiroproducts. In a promotion for his first layman movie, which was done in the late sixties, he says, "This one pre-dates the lifetime maintenance idea and is strongly anti-medical, but still contains a great number of wonderful analogies and explanations." The same could be said for almost all of B.J.'s writings. To date, the most comprehensive explanation of chiropractic by Reggie is contained on a set of ten audio cassettes that were produced in 1987 just after his return to chiropractic from Spinology. It is easily his best work and certainly the best, most systematic, audio presentation ever.

He begins the tape series, which was done live at Dr. Dave Blessing's chiropractic office, with the question, "Why should chiropractic have a philosophy?" The fact is that virtually no other profession from medicine to law to architecture has a philosophy. He explains that chiropractic does not *have* a philosophy, chiropractic *is* a philosophy. It is a philosophy of life and adjusting vertebral subluxations is an art that has grown out of that philosophy. The general purpose of philosophy, Reg submits, "is not to supply answers but to supply questions." It is interesting that one of the greatest criticisms of objective straight chiropractic philosophy is that it is dogmatic, that it is forced upon the student and the chiropractor in a catechismal manner. Some people have the impression that the straight chiropractic community teaches "it is this way or no way." Yet Reggie's presentation is anything but that. The whole thrust of his introduction in this particular tape series is that straight chiropractic, being deductive in nature, is trying to encourage people to think rather than follow what has been imposed upon them. Reg says, "The job of a teacher is not to fill the mind but to open the mind." Reggie's development of this concept is among the most important contributions to chiropractic in the last twenty years. For as much as B.J. based his philosophy on a deductive model, it was largely taught from an authoritarian viewpoint. Palmer did not encourage people to open their minds, question his authority or challenge traditionally held beliefs in light of logic. As a result, the logical approach to chiropractic was largely ignored in favor of a dogmatic approach. That approach still exists today in the form of the traditional approach to chiropractic (based on B.J.'s dogma rather than his logic) and is taught by the ICA Schools. Reggie has always wanted to change that. To him, the purpose of the philosophy is "to cause thought, to help people to follow the logic of their own understanding, to achieve a pathway of truth." His position is that induction gives us knowledge but understanding can only occur through a process of deduction.

The basis for the study of anything is to gain knowledge. Unfortunately the complexity of the universe and of the human body in particular necessitates breaking that study into manageable parts. That is the inductive method and that is why we have specialties in the health field. Even the specialty of disease treatment (medicine) is broken down into further specialties. Of course, the weakness of this approach is that it is difficult to understand something apart from its relationship of the whole.

Reg demonstrates the fallacy of "The-whole-is-equal-to-the-sum-of its-parts" theory, particularly when studying something that has invisible parts like the human body's innate intelligence.

It does not lend itself to the empirical study of induction because it is not understood by use of the senses. The fallacy of "The-whole-is-equal..." theory is not so much that the theory is incorrect but that by induction we only ever study some of the parts. Reg notes, "When you make decisions based on partial knowledge, you take a great risk." From here he logically explains the fallacy of applying the scientific method to medicine and art and shows that medicine is not a science. Reg uses medicine and the medical approach as an example of how the inductive process is applied and how it is anything but scientific. While he is explaining a technical, philosophical concept, namely induction, his presentation is anything but dry and uninteresting. He uses various analogies, stories and examples that everyone can relate to. His discussion includes the weakness of the outside-in approach to normalizing body chemistry and takes parts of his "Chemistry of Life" talk to reinforce the concept that you cannot possibly balance someone else's body chemistry when you do not know what is normal for every individual. He explains the three shortcomings of inductive reasoning as they relate to the human body:

1. We don't know enough about the human body to use induction. We only know some of the parts.
2. Even if we could look at all the parts we might still draw wrong conclusions. He uses the example that the cholesterol build up in arteries may be the result of cardiovascular disease rather than the cause of it.
3. In the living body the whole is not equal to the sum of its parts. It is undeniably more than this because there are unquantifiable factors.

It is worth noting that throughout this and all of Reggie's presentations, he never once refers to notes. Even though he spends nearly twenty minutes in this talk covering his second point, he is able to move on to his third point as if he had at least an outline in front of him. He never appears to be jumping from one subject to another. His presentation is always organized and flows logically from one topic to the next, making it easy and enjoyable for the listener. Even when he wants to add something onto a point he has already passed he does so effortlessly. In this talk, before he covers Point 3, he realizes that another example to explain Point 1 would be helpful. He reviews Point 1 as if summing up the first two points, adds on his other example and proceeds to Point 3. His ability to read the audience, be flexible in his presentation and totally recall all his material is something that is exciting to observe.

Reg then moves right into an explanation of deductive reasoning. He makes an interesting observation that the Big Idea B.J. talks about is the Major Premise. All else will follow by simple laws of logic. He makes it clear that chiropractic, as a philosophy of life, is developed by deduction. His caveat is that the primary premise must be correct and he goes to great length to give examples of how people have grown up with false assumptions as an a priori principle and from that have drawn false conclusions. The weakness of deductive reasoning is that if the premise is incorrect then the conclusions will likely be incorrect.

Reg discusses the principle of organization to explain universal intelligence using the atom as an example. He presents the analogy of finding a pocket watch as an indication of the existence of universal intelligence. He makes the point that whether you accept vitalism or mechanism depends upon which makes the most sense to your logical mind. Obviously, vitalism, and the idea that there is order and organization in the universe, is more logical to him than the idea of everything being here by random chance.

He then makes the transition from universal intelligence to innate intelligence, explaining the organization of a single cell. He also differentiates between innate and universal intelligence using B.J.'s analogy of the sun and its rays. Reg sees a clear distinction between innate intelligence and the cosmos or God. He says, "Innate intelligence does not tell you where to practice or make your mental decisions for you." One of the things that is so admirable about Reggie is his unwillingness to skirt important issues, to soften the philosophy or to avoid areas of controversy. It has probably lost him more friends than it has won him but when it comes to the message of chiropractic, it has made him the most respected chiropractor in the world. He spends a great deal of time discussing the concept of innate intelligence leading into the topic of the Triune of Life, which is the concept that encompasses the fundamental principle of chiropractic.

In discussing the third aspect of the triune, force, Reg notes that there may be other forces within the body. These forces may even be addressed by other healing arts, but chiropractic only deals with the force used by the innate intelligence of the body to organize the matter of the body. Reg clearly defines the chiropractic objective, "The purpose of chiropractic then is to maintain the uninterrupted perfection of the triune of life." Much of the information and many of the concepts that Reg explains in this series is new material, or at least material that I have never heard before. It is, however, important and I would encourage every practicing chiropractor to listen to it. I am impressed here, as always, by the fact that Reg never misspeaks. I was shocked to hear the president of a chiropractic college use the term "chiropractic treatment" in the Centennial Video. This was a third-generation chiropractor whose grandfather was a close friend of B.J. Reggie never accidentally says the wrong thing. Perhaps it is because he speaks as much as he does. Of course, you would never expect to hear him use the term "manipulate" instead of adjustment but he will never even flippantly say "innate." He always uses the term "innate intelligence" or the "intelligence of the body" or another appropriate term. In teaching chiropractic from a technical standpoint, he is always specific and precise in what he says.

Reg, then, moves into the specifics of chiropractic, what it is and what it is not. He clearly states, as he always has, what constitutes the practice of chiropractic and what does not. He does not comment as to whether a chiropractor should or should not do other things, but emphasizes that they are not chiropractic. At this point, he discusses what may be the most important idea of the entire presentation. That is "the qualities of a good chiropractor." He maintains that the primary quality is not a commitment to the care of the patient but a commitment to serve the principle. Many chiropractors stray from straight chiropractic on this point. The patient has many needs in the physical realm as well as in the emotional, the spiritual and in other realms. If the chiropractor attempts to care for the whole person, the objective of correcting vertebral subluxations is lessened. There is no doubt that there are many valuable things that can be done to and for a person. On occasions, treating their symptoms may even be one of them. Surely a person in the terminal stages of a painful illness wants and deserves some relief. The chiropractor who dissipates his time and talent, however, lessens his ability to be the best chiropractor he can be. The second quality of a good chiropractor is sensitivity. Being sensitive to the needs of the patient and the desires of the patient's innate intelligence. Reg emphasizes that determining the innate needs and desires of the body when it comes to the spine and the body's desire to correct subluxation is an educated function. This is especially important in the muscle palpation technique that Reggie developed. The chiropractor analyzes what the innate intelligence of the patient's body is trying to do using the musculature system to correct a subluxation. A good chiropractor recognizes that each patient is different, in fact each subluxation is different and has its own special needs.

Chiropractic first aid is not a part of the chiropractor's care and there may be times when the patient who is in pain is not ready or able to accept the chiropractor's force. Often that is when the patient believes that he needs an adjustment the most. Reg is clear that our job is not to please the patient by trying to give him relief. He stresses the need to communicate to the patient the importance of what we do. Most of us are not communicating properly to patients, not getting them to truly understand what we do. He discusses the art of active conversation, getting patients involved in the learning process rather than being an innocent and often ignorant bystander.

Reggie emphasizes at the outset of the presentation that chiropractic really has very little to do with correcting subluxations, that it is really a philosophy of life. No where does he make that more clear than when he begins to discuss universal laws and the importance of understanding and living according to them, in his discussion of cause and effect, he points out that very little in life is a matter of luck and he relates this to chiropractic practice. Succeeding in practice does not depend on luck as a chiropractor, you cannot change the effect unless you address the cause. His message is that each chiropractor has to take responsibility for his own success or failure because the cause is within.

Reg spends a good deal of time on this tape discussing limitations of matter, and rightfully so, since too many chiropractors do not realize the limitations that are placed upon the body. Many have an unrealistic image of what the innate intelligence can do. This particular concept was important to Reggie's understanding. When he realized the body could not cure everything, he then had a basis for a philosophy about what the body can do, i.e., work better without subluxation, which has become his primary message. An unrealistic idea of limitations of matter also causes many chiropractors to begin to think that if the body cannot heal itself, then they should heal it. They fail to realize that if the body cannot heal itself, then nobody else can heal it, least of all their finite educated mind. Reg then covers the subject of symptoms, logically explaining why we cannot depend on them as a barometer of health and why the chiropractor does not address them.

A considerable portion of this series is spent on questions and answers and there is probably no other chiropractor in the world who is better at this teaching format. It is obvious that Reggie enjoys a good question and answer period. He encourages questions and allows at least some time for this type of exchange in most of his talks. He has such a command of his subject matter that he is entirely confident he has an answer for any question. He admits that his answer might not be satisfactory to the questioner, but it always satisfies his own criteria which is that the answer be logical. He enjoys succeeding and admits that being able to field any and every question gives one a sense of succeeding. You know that every individual walking out of your talk has understood what you have said, within their abilities. That does not mean that they necessarily have accepted, it but they have understood it.

As a teacher, Reg enjoys student's questions. Any good teacher does. When a student asks questions, not for clarification, but good, probing, insightful questions, it means the student is thinking. Getting his listeners to think is his most important objective and when a student asks this type of question he knows he has accomplished his objective, at least in one person.

One of the first questions that Reg is asked in this presentation involves chiropractors who address the cause of vertebral subluxations. He explains that not only is it difficult to know what all these contributing factors may be for any one individual but it is simply impossible to address many, if not all of those factors. To succeed, a person must be focused. No matter how valuable it is to run around and pick up banana peels, it dissipates the chiropractor's energies, especially when there are others trained to do it, whose job it is. In responding, he gives a glimpse of himself that most in the mixing aspect of this profession do not know. They view him as a radical straight who hates mixers and who would drive them all out of practice if given the chance. That may well have been the image he portrayed twenty years ago when the straight movement was fighting for its professional life, but this is a kinder, gentler Reggie Gold. After explaining why he would not address the cause, he says, "however, I will not condemn somebody else who does... an individual chiropractor should behave according to his or her conscience. You are not just a chiropractor, you are a human being." He does warn his listeners though, that "compassion can draw you out of chiropractic." While he does not judge those who want to help solve world problems other than or in addition to the correction of subluxation, he makes his position clear. "My job... is to serve in two capacities both of which are as a chiropractor. The easy one is working to locate, identify and introduce a force for the correction of vertebral subluxation. The second encompasses the other, that is, to share with the world my chiropractic philosophy."

In spite of his being a kinder, gentler Reggie, in the next talk in this series he takes off on some of the techniques that chiropractors use that are questionably chiropractic. Reggie has no problems with someone who wants to mix, as long as they do it in a legitimate, acceptable and competent manner. He still has no time for chiropractors who would defraud their patients with some sort of system or procedure that has no scientific or rational basis.

As far as Reggie is concerned, it is the practitioner's prerogative to practice an accepted therapeutic method and mix it with chiropractic. However, if you are going to make up something new and call it chiropractic, it must have some kind of logical, philosophical and/or scientific basis to it. It appears that at least some of the systems are merely a means for entrepreneurial chiropractors to put on technique seminars at tremendous cost to students who have been cheated out of a decent education in chiropractic college and feel they are incompetent to adjust spines in practice.

Reggie's real concern about many of these techniques is not their worthlessness but the fact that they do work on symptoms to some degree if only as a placebo effect. In fact, that was his earliest criticism of Concept Therapy and what led to his split with D.E. Many of these procedures have the psychological effect of getting rid of the patient's symptoms. Unfortunately, if those symptoms are caused by a life-threatening medical problem, then the chiropractor may be doing the patient a grave disservice by relieving their symptoms. Contrast that with the true objective of straight chiropractic, which allows the body's inner wisdom to normalize function. If and when the symptoms go away, it is because the body has decided that they should go away. It is not the result of mind games played by the doctor on the patient's educated mind. It doesn't matter if it works or not. Our job is to work with the perfect innate wisdom of the body, not to use our imperfect educated brain or the patient's imperfect educated brain to try to run the body or to establish what we think is right for it. Every time we do that we send a clear message to the patient and to everyone around us and them that is directly opposed to what we want the world to hear and come to understand.

The thrust of much of Reggie's presentation is teaching chiropractors to teach chiropractic philosophy to the world. With all the confusion as to our professional identity, chiropractors stealing medical therapies, medicine stealing chiropractic, Reggie's message is clear and simple. We have a philosophy that no one can steal. It is based upon deductive reasoning and the world needs to hear it. Not only do they need to hear it but in acting in accordance with it they will be better off and you will be a successful chiropractor.

One very important question that Reg addresses and one that really frustrates many straight chiropractors relates to the benefits of chiropractic care. If we cannot or should not relate chiropractic to disease relief, cure or prevention, how can we convince the public of the benefits of regular chiropractic care for life? His response is that every aspect of human physiology and function in life is dependent upon the nerve system. If there is vertebral subluxation none of the body's functions can occur as they should. Your health will improve with chiropractic care because every aspect of life is better without nerve interference. That we can promise people. What we can never promise or imply is that any particular improvement will occur.

The last question Reg addresses in this tape series is very apropos. Earlier, Reg stated that educating people is more important than adjusting patients. This question challenges that statement. Reg responds that he is bothered by the self-serving, yuppie generation that is only interested in making money. We have a philosophy worth sharing, one of the few. Our purpose in chiropractic should be to help people. Education is more important because that is what will change the world. Learning to adjust is not that difficult, medical doctors and even physical therapists are learning it. Changing peoples' perception of life is much more difficult, much more important and much more of a challenge. As Reg ends this ten-cassette series, he leaves the listeners with this challenge and the promise that the second ten-tape series will give the chiropractor the tools he or she needs to educate patients.

His second series of tapes is really a continuation of the philosophy despite the fact that its focus is on practical application. The philosophy is not what you do but what you think. He returns to the theme that chiropractic involves an entire philosophy of life based upon a major premise and a deductive approach to thinking. Historically, it began as a treatment for one disease (deafness) and evolved into a cure for many diseases but eventually a philosophy was formed around it and the philosophy is what became important. If you practice the art but ignore the principles of chiropractic, it is not chiropractic. It is physical medicine, osteopathy or some other therapy. From the very outset of this series, Reggie lays the groundwork for his entire presentation. A body with no interference in the nerve system works better than one with interference. That is chiropractic. Further, how do you know that statement is true? Why does one accept it? Simply because it makes sense. It does not necessitate research or induction or a tremendous exercise of faith. It just makes sense. His entire presentation, not just in this series but really in everything he says, can be distilled into these two points:

1. Everybody is better off without vertebral subluxations.
2. This fact can be demonstrated to any person who will use logic and common sense as a reference point.

Chiropractic bases its practice and success on a principle, which is true and works in every case. Medicine, on the other hand, bases its practice on percentages, nine out of ten get better with this procedure so the odds are with the patient, at least in most cases. The first aspect of practice discussion for Reg is getting his listener to see that the use of diagnosis in the practice of chiropractic is illogical. He makes it clear that he is not trying to build million-dollar practices. He does not care how much money a chiropractor makes. What he does care about is that whole communities be full of unsubluxated people and the only way that will happen is if chiropractors have the ability and the tools to teach people about chiropractic.

He attacks the concept of Report of Findings. He believes that a chiropractor who does a report of findings cannot ever get the patient on the right track. If you are explaining the "cause" of the patient's complaint and your program of care, the patient is going to assume that the program is for the relief of that problem. Consequently, to try to get them to make the transition somewhere else along the line to regular, lifetime, maintenance care is a virtual impossibility. This concept, which started as a practice building procedure many years ago, has, in Reggie's estimation, done more to inhibit the building of a true chiropractic practice than anything else in the history of our profession. When people went to chiropractors in the first half of this century, they were usually given The Big Idea by the chiropractor and told they would need to "take" adjustments for the rest of their life. With the advent of the Report of Findings, chiropractic became a procedure for a problem or its cause for a prescribed period of time. Instead of a Report of Findings, Reg advocates bringing both the patient and their spouse into the office and explaining what you do. The important thing is that you do not alter your system, you do not under any circumstances compromise your principles. If it means not accepting some patients and losing a few dollars then so be it. Living and practicing according to a set of principles is much more important then making money. People will be attracted to someone who is committed to the validity of their practice. In fact, as much as Reggie's presentation revolves around demonstrating the logic of chiropractic to people, he admits that people are first turned on by your dedication and enthusiasm.

In presenting chiropractic to a new patient (and spouse), Reggie again recommends a concept called active conversation. This involves interacting with the patient in order to get them to tell you about their work, their life, their problems and activities and then relating chiropractic to those areas of the patients' life to show them how regular chiropractic care can help them excel in all of those areas. This type of approach represents a dramatic departure from the straight approach of the previous decade. Most straight chiropractors have discouraged any type of discourse with the patient except for the doctor's monologue during which he explains what he is going to do as a straight chiropractor and what he is not going to do. Reggie believes that this approach has fallen largely on deaf ears, often deafened by the patients' concern for their physical problem. By getting patients to open up and join the dialogue, they will be much more receptive to what chiropractic can do for them and their unique needs.

Reg spends a considerable amount of time explaining how to convert your practice. He draws an analogy between quitting smoking and accepting patients for back pain, what he calls patch-up care. In both, he says you must make the decision to quit and then do it. There must be commitment that you will not accept patients who do not want lifetime, family, maintenance care. You must burn your bridges and may even turn a few patients away to make it work. At this point he introduces what I think is one of the most unique and innovative ideas in building a family, maintenance-care practice. He calls it the "You be the Judge" program. The chiropractor, after he or she has explained chiropractic to both parents, offers to accept the entire family for regular chiropractic care, for one month, completely free of charge. If after that time the family sees no improvement in their health, life or relationship, then they can quit and it has cost them absolutely nothing. If they have seen the benefits of chiropractic care, they can sign up for the regular, yearly fee program (which Reg recommends). Reg tells the story of one of his seminar attendees who moved into a new town and tried this program, signing up forty families. Twenty of these families ultimately signed up for yearly care at the end of the month. After two months in practice he was seeing ninety patients a week.

Reg emphasizes the difference between the medical model and the chiropractic model. At this point in the tape series, he discusses the importance of building your practice in the chiropractic model rather than in the medical one, with special emphasis given to the area of patient education. The medical doctor does nothing in the area of patient education. He frankly does not want the patient to know anything about what he is doing except for the purpose of building confidence in himself or insuring cooperation. It is not necessary nor is it helpful to his care. The chiropractor, on the other hand, knows that every decision a patient needs to make regarding his or her health, except for one, can and should be made by the patient. (The one decision of course is whether his or her spine needs to be adjusted or not.)

Reg divides his patient education program into four phases. Phase One includes the patient orientation, the interview and the dialogue that takes place between the chiropractor and the patient and spouse. Phase Two is the reinforcement of this information through lecture on what Reg prefers to call "Chiropractic Night." These are done at least once a month. It should be noted that these are not a substitution for a patient orientation which is custom tailored to the patient and is in dialogue format. The lay lecture is for patients to bring their friends and loved ones to, to introduce them to chiropractic. The message is the same but the examples are general. It does not have to be different than the orientation since repetition is the best teacher. Reggie is a strong proponent of repetition. He often notes that people have to be told again and again that they are always better off without subluxations.

Phase Three is the continued dialogue between the chiropractor and the patient during daily visits. Phase Four is a continuing education series of six lectures on six consecutive weeks. Reg suggests that the first one be on the difference between inductive and deductive reasoning so that patients are better able to think from an ADIO perspective. The series should also include the triune of life, innate matter, innate intelligence and innate force. This will help people to change their entire way of thinking and will really begin to make a difference in their lives and in the world.

Reg spends a considerable amount of time in this series on the issue of malpractice. In his clear and logical way he tears apart what he calls, the "tissue of lies" that the mixing element of our profession has told concerning malpractice, especially regarding the necessity for diagnosis. Failing to diagnose or diagnosing incorrectly when treating a medical condition is the greatest cause of malpractice. However, choosing not to diagnose, choosing not to treat a medical condition and so informing the patient is a safe and simple approach to the practice of chiropractic. In fact, it is the safest, most enjoyable way to practice.

Toward the end of the series, Reggie gets into some practical ways to build the practice or more appropriately to see more patients.

He again makes it clear that he is not a practice builder and he does not really care to make chiropractors rich or successful. He wants to enable them to get their entire community under regular chiropractic maintenance care. He discusses what your waiting room should look like, how you should talk to patients on a regular basis and public-relation endeavors that will expose more of the community to life-enhancing chiropractic care.

One of the practical aspects of his tape series is in helping the chiropractor to answer questions asked by patients. Reg contends that just answering a patient's question without giving him the principle behind that question is similar to giving him a fish rather than teaching him to fish. If patients understand the principles behind the questions, then not only will they be equipped to answer the question themselves but other questions of a similar nature will not have to be asked. Most important, patients will have a principle to apply to all aspects of their lives. The principle of cause and effect is a perfect example. Chiropractic happens to be cause oriented, correcting vertebral subluxations, a cause of DISEASE. If the patient understands the cause and effect principle, he can apply it to other aspects of his life. This particular principle is important because it enables people to realize that they are in control of their lives or should be in control. If there were no relationship between cause and effect, our lives would be a matter of chance.

One of Reggie's greatest communication skills is his ability to draw analogies that help the listener understand various aspects of the chiropractic philosophy. He has the ability to weave humorous stories and jokes into his presentation without disrupting his message. This is due, in part, to the fact that his anecdotes have a purpose, they always emphasize a philosophical concept. It is interesting to note that his earlier talks are consistently laced with these analogies, where his later talks seem to have fewer and fewer. This indicates the evolution of his understanding of the chiropractic philosophy. An analogy's purpose is to make a principle or idea that is not clear more understandable to the listener. The analogies have lessened over time because Reg has brought his presentation of chiropractic to such a simple, logical, easily understood level that analogies are not as necessary. His latest talks could be given almost without any analogies. The few analogies that he does draw are almost there for humor or to entertain the listener. His explanation of chiropractic is so simple that further explanation is not necessary.

One of the first lay lectures of Reggie's that I was able to listen to begins with the story of Billy Ryan, the little boy who, while lying terminally ill in the hospital was adjusted by Dr. William Werner. He had been in a coma for four days and the medical resident of the hospital said Billy would be dead in forty-eight hours. The morning after the adjustment, he was out of the coma. Within four weeks he was home and thirty years later he was still under chiropractic care. Reg's message was that there was still something that could be done after medicine failed. Reg goes on to explain why the boy got well and why he got sick. He explains right away, "It was a miracle but not a miracle of chiropractic. Reg makes what is one of his earliest and most quoted statements still applicable almost thirty years later, "Chiropractic never cured anybody of anything." He explains that "the job of the chiropractor is not to cure."

Reg's emphasis at this point (in 1970) was not that chiropractic gets sick people well, but that the body has a better chance of healing without nerve interference. Reg has always stressed that the body does the healing, but along with that, he began to note that subluxation should be corrected because it, in and of itself, is bad. He makes his point with the example of treating a headache with aspirin, "... and it comes back. But even if it didn't come back, would you want to go through life with vital nerves pinched off just as long as they don't cause pain?" His major emphasis, however, was still on chiropractic as a prevention for disease.

Reggie's Analogies

In the early years, before Reg had perfected and simplified his presentation, the stories, analogies and case histories abound. In this series, they include the following:

1. An army and the body. An army, to be effective, must be organized, must have a general and must have a communication system. If the communication system is interfered with, the army will not function in a coordinated manner. The same is true with the body and its innate intelligence and the nerve system, respectively.

2. Uncle Charlie's cold. Uncle Charlie comes to visit a family with four children and plays with each of them equally. One gets it and has it for a week, another for two weeks and another ends up with pneumonia, while the fourth child doesn't get it at all. The fact that all people do not respond the same way to the same virus refutes the germ theory.

3. Pain is an expensive alarm system within your body. You would not cut the wires of the alarm in your house if it went off in the middle of the night. Yet, people take pain killers to do just that to the alarm systems in their bodies.

4. Electronic Short Circuit. An interference in the nerve system is analogous to a short circuit in an electrical system.

5. The Man falling off the Empire State Building. (This one always gets a laugh!) At every floor, he says "so far I feel fine." However, by the time the first symptom appears, he is dead. People ignore their health for years, saying "I feel fine and by the time the first symptom appears, it is too late.

6. Body cells are replaced every seven years. That means that every seven years you have an entirely new body. This example prompts his humorous statement, "That means if you've been married for 21 years, you are already on your third wife."

In a 1970 talk, Reg uses good, old fashion logic. He asked a D.E. group, "Does anyone believe that chiropractic is a part of medicine?" Of course, back comes the resounding answer, "No!" He deduces, then, that if medicine is the ail encompassing treatment of disease, then, chiropractic must be something else. He proceeds to explain chiropractic has nothing to do with disease. In this same talk, he does his well-known blackboard drawing with the D.C. (Doctor of Chiropractic) on one side and the D.T. (Doctor of Therapy) on the other, which includes all the therapies (including those practiced by chiropractors) and spinal manipulation therapy.

He makes a very important point here (remember this is 1970). "Chiropractic is the adjustment of the spine... for the correction of the cause of DIS-EASE, not diseases." Chiropractic opens up the nerve channels. Trying to make a physiological change in the patient makes whatever you are doing a therapy. Sadly, the leadership of that particular group has spent the last twenty-six years teaching that chiropractors correct the cause of disease.

Reggie also explains in some of these early talks how diagnosis is totally irrational if you are practicing straight chiropractic. This was at least four years before the acceptance of the CCE. He says, "In chiropractic, we have no use for diagnosis whatsoever, absolutely none. Why? Because we are not going to treat diseases... It does not relate to the treatment of disease...We do one thing only... We examine the spine to determine whether the placement of the spine is offering an insult to the nervous system... We introduce a force." Chiropractors by the thousands were hearing this message in 1970. Why did they all sell out when CCE came along? By selling out I do not mean to imply that many simply gave into the power of the CCE and blindly followed their dictates. These people actually tried to justify them. Everyone in that meeting agreed with Reggie. Yet, six years later, that same group was proclaiming his approach as irrational chiropractic.

During this particular D.E. seminar in July of 1970, Reg gave some of the greatest talks he has ever given. He expanded the ADIO philosophy further than anyone had ever heard him before on a public platform. He has apparently not shared that level of his philosophy with a group of people since that time, focusing more on simplifying the philosophy. Those D.E. seminars in the early seventies were very special. More dedicated chiropractors gathered together there than at any place, at any time since B.J.'s old Lyceums. And these chiropractors were dedicated to service, not to making money.

Reg had literally hours to share with the audience both from the platform and during late night informal sessions. Besides chiropractic philosophy, he got into the philosophy of giving, of loving and of being "tuned into station WGOD."

In making his chiropractic message simpler and more easily understood, he no longer takes the opportunity to share his personal philosophy of life with chiropractors. Occasionally, glimpses of it will come through, especially at Sherman Lyceums when he is "preaching to the faithful," but for the most part, he gives the simple, basic chiropractic message. Reggie used some great analogies, stories and examples which include the following.

1. Darkness and light and disease and health. This analogy is one of the most important explanations of a chiropractic principle that has ever been shared with humanity. I wrote an entire book on health for lay people, *Enhance Your Life Experience,* based upon this "Reganalogy." Darkness is the absence of light. You cannot hold it, create it or sweep it out of the room. It simply does not exist in the presence of light. Similarly, disease is a manifestation of the absence of health. Chiropractors do not try to get rid of disease, they restore health.

2. Respecting the educated mind versus the innate brain. We respect the educated mind because it can supposedly determine how much insulin an individual body needs. Yet, that very mind was a peanut butter and jelly sandwich yesterday and it is only able to think today because the innate intelligence converted the sandwich into brain tissue. We should have more respect for the innate wisdom and allow it to determine the insulin needs.

3. Chow Mein and Ptomaine. Reggie uses the analogy of two people who go to a Chinese restaurant, order Chow Mein but get ptomaine poisoning. One manifests symptoms, but the other does not. Which one is actually sick? The body may very well be getting rid of a poison when it manifests unpleasant symptoms. That does not mean it is sick. On the contrary, it means it

is healthy. A body working properly may flush poisons from the system by vomiting and diarrhea.

4. Scientific proof of chiropractic. Asking the scientific community (which in the area of health is medicine) to evaluate the efficiency of chiropractic is like asking Cadillac people to give you an unbiased evaluation of Mercedes Benz.

5. Laws of the Universe and the Laws of Life. The laws of the universe, for example gravity, are immutable and unswerving. You cannot violate them. You must live within them. Similarly, the laws of life, for example, innate intelligence and its expression in the body are also immutable. Chiropractic attempts to enable the individual to live within those laws.

6. Understanding normal and average. Reg tells the story of the man who throws up after every meal and believes that is normal just because he does it. In explaining the danger of this concept, he uses the story to emphasize that we cannot allow the patient's educated brain to establish what is normal.

7. Building a large, successful practice and patients being healthy. Many chiropractors want to know how to build a successful practice without giving up all the things that make them a failure. Similarly, patients want to know the same about health. They neither want to give up the things that keep them from being healthy nor do the things that make them healthy, like getting their spines checked every week.

8. The Indian and the Feather. Some of Reggie's analogies are humorous, some even border on silly. He uses the story about the Indian who sleeps on a feather one night, the next morning he wakes up with a stiff neck and a headache and says, "White man foolish, feather not soft for sleeping." Similarly, people will get one or two adjustments and think that is enough and that regular care is not needed.

9. Knowing where you are and where you are going. In explaining the idea of changing your chiropractic objective, Reggie uses the analogy of following a map. You must first know where you are before you can determine where you are going. Similarly, we must understand our thinking and where it is incorrect before we can philosophically get to the right place.

10. Jar of Nuts. Reg gave a talk at a Palmer homecoming about doing whatever is necessary to get the chiropractic message across to people and build a practice. All the while he was shaking ajar of mixed nuts. By the end of the talk, the largest nuts had risen to the top. His message, to get to the top you have to be a big nut.

11. Finding a Wristwatch. The organization of a watch with all its intricacies bespeaks an intelligent person who designed and organized it. Similarly, the body bespeaks organization and hence, also an intelligence. This analogy was actually first used by Henry David Thoreau.

12. Albert Schweitzer. The famous doctor said the most difficult part of bringing medical care to the natives was getting them to give up their superstitions. Similarly, our greatest job in chiropractic is to get people to give up their superstitions about medicine and health.

13. A Light Bulb. A rheostat reduces the quantity and the quality of the light emitted from the bulb. Similarly, a vertebral subluxation reduces the quantity and quality of the mental impulse.

Reg also tells the story of Bill Allen, the US Army Colonel, who was diagnosed as "terminal" with cancer but received chiropractic care at the B.J. Palmer Chiropractic Research Clinic and got completely well. He later became a chiropractor and practiced many years. Reg tells the story in response to a medical doctor who challenged that no one had ever recovered from cancer under chiropractic care.

In January 1971, Reggie shared with a D.E. audience the 1966 article, from *Life* magazine, on the Russian Siamese Twins who while sharing the same body got sick at different times. The story has since been picked up by various groups. Koren Publication has produced a pamphlet around the *Life* magazine article. Other analogies and explanations from this talk include:

1. DNA repairing itself. DNA that has been damaged by some universal force actually has some intelligent, self-repair mechanism, describing what we chiropractors know as innate intelligence. Reg shares this information from scientific sources.

2. The inadequacies of science. Science cannot explain or understand limitless time and space. It just accepts them on faith. Similarly, we cannot explain or understand the innate intelligence of the body, but we accept it and what it can do.

3. Organization of matter. A piece of chalk manifests organization that keeps the matter together. If it were not for the principle of organization, the energy in that chalk could destroy the world with an atomic explosion.

In a 1972 lay lecture, Reg uses the following now familiar analogies:

1. The Common Cold Cure. In explaining the foolishness of the medical approach to finding causes for disease rather than looking within the body at its own inborn healing ability, he uses the example of research being done to find a cure for the common cold. The medical approach is to search for the cure in the fetus of a whale under the arctic ice cap. By way of contrast, the chiropractor does not believe that mankind was cursed with this horrible affliction, the cold, and that the only cure for it was hidden in a whale in the arctic. The cold is not an affliction but the manifestation of an absence of proper function in the human body. (It may also well be a manifestation of proper function in the body.)

2. The Piece of Steak. This explanation of the fact that it is the liv-

ing body that heals is so simple and logical, yet it emphasizes a point that too few of the public understand. If you cut a piece of steak, put iodine and a bandage on it and give it a shot of penicillin, it still will not heal. Therefore, those things have nothing to do with the healing of the body. It is life that heals. A living body heals itself, a dead piece of steak does not. I personally used this analogy for many years in my lay lecture.

3. The Traffic Light. B.J. often said, "If you use chiropractic to get you well, you should use it to keep you well." At this point in his philosophical evolution, Reg still emphasized that getting well was only a part of chiropractic care and that patients needed to continue with chiropractic care. He uses the analogy of putting up a traffic light at a dangerous intersection. You do not take the traffic light down after there are no longer any accidents. While Reg no longer presents chiropractic as a means of getting people well, this was a excellent analogy in 1972. It could be adapted for today, using the idea that lights maintain a "healthy" flow of traffic. You would not take a light down just to see if traffic could take care of itself without any direction or control. We know that innate intelligence uses the nerve system to direct and control our *body* functions. Why would you want to see if you could do without that control?

At Sherman College, in 1975, and at other speaking engagements, Reg shared the following:

1. Standing outside a movie theater on Saturday night. Reg challenges those chiropractors who believe they are doing a good job at getting patients into the office to see how few people coming out of theater on a Saturday night are actually patients.

2. Knowing the body's needs. Cast your thought down to one little cell in your liver. What are its needs at this moment? The greatest educated mind in the world does not know the needs of a single, little cell in the body.

3. Ohio State Penitentiary Research. Convicts were implanted with cancer cells. Not surprisingly, those with a previous history of cancer again developed cancer. Interestingly, though, the other convicts did not develop cancer. In fact, their bodies actually rejected the injected cancer cells indicating that the body has an inborn ability to fight cancer.

4. Four levels of chiropractic care. Reggie developed and presented the idea of continually trying to upgrade the patient's level. The levels (from highest to lowest) are:

    1. Being subluxation free
    2. Prevention and health maintenance
    3. Getting rid of disease (chiropractic gets sick people well)
    4. Musculoskeletal condition

5. Termites in the kitchen. A couple of termites don't do much damage but over the years they multiply and destroy the framework of the house. So that one day you unsuspectingly walk across the kitchen floor and it collapses below you. Subluxations are like termites. The time to correct them is as soon as they occur.

6. Body designed to live 120-150 years. The fact is there are pockets of people in the world who do live to that age, therefore we must conclude that the body is designed to last at least that length of time.

7. Breaking your arm for free. No one would have someone break their arm even if it were for free. No one wants a broken arm. Similarly, no one will receive chiropractic care just because it is free or inexpensive. Chiropractic has to be made desirable to people.

8. Light and darkness, life and death. A corpse does not have death, it has an absence of life. A partial absence of life is called DIS-EASE. Chiropractors restore life to a body that is partially missing it.

9. Man walking on his hands because he never tried using his feet.

People are afraid to change even though it may be easier. It is much easier to practice straight chiropractic than the complicated mixing/diagnosing/treating approach. But many are afraid to try it.

10. Being lost while traveling in a car. Rather than stopping for directions, we often just drive faster and faster, and often in the wrong direction. The chiropractic profession is going in the wrong direction (toward medicine) and appears to be traveling at breakneck speed to get there.

11. Blaming sickness on old age and the weather. The arthritis in the left leg cannot be old age. The right leg is just as old. Further, we are all exposed to the same weather so the aches and pains cannot be due to that.

In a lay lecture in 1978, Reg used the following:

1. Life is like a candle. This is one of Reggie's shortest and oldest, yet it still has impact. A candle bums brightly all the way to the end, flickers once or twice and goes out. Life should be that way too. Unfortunately, most people flicker all through their life and never really bum brightly.

2. Surgeons and masks. During his anti-medicine period, Reg used the joke that surgeons wore masks for the same reason that Jesse James did. But aside from the sarcasm, the idea that a mask with as he says "bloody great holes in it," could stop a bacteria or vims is foolish.

3. Forgetting to wind your wristwatch. How fortunate we are to have an innate intelligence to keep our heart running. We who forget to wind our watch would forget to wind our heart at night and not wake up in the morning.

4. The development of a baby. Reg's explanation of how the innate

intelligence of the body "builds" a baby from two half-cells is almost a classic. Anyone who listens to his logic and detail of the order, organization and beauty of the formation of the body has to realize that there is a wisdom that can run this body for a lifetime.

5. <u>Driving with the brake on</u>. It can be done and perhaps not ever noticed but once the emergency brake is removed, the car has more "energy." Similarly, people may come to the office thinking that they are healthy and that there is nothing wrong with them. Then when they have received chiropractic adjustments for a while, they realize that they really were not reaching their full potential and experiencing all that life had to offer.

Reggie made his unofficial entrance back into chiropractic at a talk at Jay Kaufman's office in Matamoras, Pennsylvania, in 1986. The title of Reg's talk that day was "Give Me One Good Reason." It was, of course, one good reason to go to a chiropractor. The talk was not much different than many of Reg's previous talks. It was the title of the talk that set the tone for the thrust of his presentation from this point on. Reg's talks for the lay person would, from that point on be directed toward finding the "one good reason" that would appeal to every person on the face of the earth. Those without back problems, those without headaches, every person sick or well needs one good reason for going to the chiropractor on a regular basis. Reg wanted to simplify the message and make it attractive to every one of those people and then teach chiropractors how they could do it also. He used the analogy of a rabbit brain generator in this talk although he had used it many times before.

In the analogy he explains that terminals can be hooked up to the brain of a rabbit to run a radio. He stated that a large, eastern university had actually performed this experiment. Results showed that while the radio ran well, the set up did drain the life from the rabbit.

In the 1987, ten-cassette Philosophy Series mentioned earlier, Reg uses the following pearls:

1. Comparison between the universe and the human body. The universe demonstrates order, organization and a cause and effect relationship. Nothing happens by chance or luck. Similarly, the human body is an organized entity that demonstrates intelligence.

2. Railroad Crossing guard who doesn't tell the whole truth. At the inquest over a night time accident, the guard swears that he waved his lantern to oncoming cars. What he failed to testify, however, was that he had forgotten to light his lantern. Similarly, chiropractors who fail to tell the whole story about chiropractic, what it can do and what it cannot do, are deceiving their patients, and more importantly, causing them to experience less than the full life they deserve. A part of the truth is not the truth.

3. The Ant on the Rembrandt. What the ant sees is only part of the whole, and hence, is not a very accurate description of the painting. What we know and understand about the body is seen from a similarly limited view and hence, can not accurately describe its overall function.

4. Coyotes in Arizona. Man in his educated attempt to improve his environment has often made it worse. All the coyotes were killed off to save farm animals. However, it upset the balance of nature causing an overabundance of rodents which are the natural prey of the coyote. Coyotes had to be raised and released to try to bring back the balance. The best that man can do is leave the environment alone and begin to adapt himself to it.

5. Flies and the garbage can. This is one of Reg's oldest, and in my opinion, very best analogies. No one blames the flies for the pile of garbage they gather on. What good would it do to kill the flies but not clean the garbage pail? Germs feed on sick bodies because they are unable to set up housekeeping in healthy ones. In later years, he also used the example of a dead bird in the road being eaten by maggots. No one concludes that the mag-

gots jumped up and killed a bird.

6. Dropping a dime in the Pacific Ocean. Reggie uses Archimedes' principle of the mass displacement of fluid to explain that if the principle of chiropractic care is correct, (i.e., if correcting vertebral subluxations enables the body to work better), it is correct in every person even though, like dropping a coin in the ocean, the change may not always be measurable.

7. Taking aspirin and taking ten minutes off your life. In explaining the cause and effect principle, Reg uses the often quoted possibility that each aspirin reduces your life span by ten minutes. Unfortunately, people do not realize this. He suggests that it would be far better if they dropped dead for ten minutes right after they took the aspirin, then came back to life. The point, of course, is we do not know how much we are losing but everything we do for the body has an effect, either positive or negative.

8. Ptomaine instead of Chow Mein. This one is almost a classic in explaining how symptoms may not necessarily be bad. It was mentioned earlier, however, in this series Reg expands upon the analogy. The body could be manifesting vomiting and diarrhea as a means of getting rid of poisons. Reg is quick to point out, however, that symptoms may also be an indication that something is wrong. In previous talks, his emphasis had been on symptoms being good. In this talk, it changes to the fact that we just can not know whether a symptom is good or bad. He notes that this is a good reason why chiropractors should not use symptoms as a criteria.

9. The Amoebae and the pin. Even a one-celled organism, like an amoebae, if alive will respond to an outside stimulation and attempt to adapt itself to it, thus explaining the third sign of life. He then explains the chiropractor's role in enabling the body to adapt.

10. Glass of ocean water and universal and innate intelligence. B.J.

used the sun and the sun's rays to explain the relationship between innate and universal intelligence. Reggie uses the ocean and ocean water in a glass to describe this relationship. Universal intelligence and innate intelligence are both principles of organization. They have some of the same characteristics and some different ones. Similarly, ocean water and a glass of ocean water have the same characteristic (e.g., chemical content) and also some different ones (e.g., shape).

11. Heart attack "victim". This example shows the foolishness of depending on how you feel to determine how you are. People with no symptoms whatsoever, who feel perfectly fine, drop dead of heart attacks or are told they have some terrible disease, including AIDS.

In the follow-up set of audio tapes, the practical application of the philosophy, Reg uses a few additional analogies including:

12. A carpenter has to hit a nail that has a sharp point to drive it through. Similarly, the objective straight chiropractor has to come to point, to focus all of his or her energies on one thing to have an impact upon society.

13. Sticking your finger in the ocean. This analogy goes along with the one above. For some people, the impact that they have upon society is like the change in the ocean after they have withdrawn their finger. In chiropractic, we have so much ability to have so much effect upon people and the world but we must "come to point" as Reg says, "to focus on doing one thing and doing it well."

14. Light bulb on the forehead. This one began much earlier but it paints such a good picture for the patient that it has stood the test of time. If we all had bulbs in our foreheads that turned on whenever we were subluxated, we could go to the chiropractor whenever our bulbs were on. Unfortunately, we do not have such a bulb. Consequently, we cannot know when we are sub-

luxated and we need to be checked regularly by our chiropractor.

In 1988, Reg was using the following stories and analogies:

1. Tying a piece of string around your aorta. As the non-straight aspect of the profession clamored for more acceptance, everyone was asking for research to prove the effectiveness of chiropractic care. Reg used this simple little example to demonstrate the logic of chiropractic care, regardless of the absence or presence of research. If you tie a string around your aorta, would that cause you any noticeable problem? Perhaps. Perhaps not. However, would your body be better off without the piece of string tied around your aorta? Absolutely. Another similar analogy is putting a rubber band snugly around a finger. When would be the intelligent time to take it off? Waiting until gangrene or blood poisoning occurred would be foolish. In this way, Reg demonstrates that common sense says have vertebral subluxations corrected as soon as you can, regardless of whether diagnosed medical conditions have been "proven" to be caused by them or not.

2. Insurance and chiropractic. In explaining why insurance companies and the government should not pay for true chiropractic care, Reg demonstrates that chiropractic is health care, something done to stay healthy. The government does not reimburse you for going to a health food store to buy naturally grown food stuffs. Insurance companies do not reimburse you for your dues at a health club. Why should they be expected to pay for chiropractic care if chiropractic care is not a therapeutic approach to the treatment of certain diseases? In 1988 this was a true statement. In 1997 some insurance companies deduct some of the premium for regular attendance at a health club.

At a 1991 Sherman Lyceum, Reg clearly set forth the distinguishing characteristic of chiropractic. He explained that our philosophy does not make us unique and really does not even define chiropractic. There are many religions and healing arts with a vitalistic philosophy, many of which have as their basis a universal intelligence. But for chiropractic, that philosophy is coupled with a practice objective. The idea of correcting vertebral subluxations to enable the body's innate intelligence to be better expressed is the chiropractic objective. That is what makes chiropractic unique. In that context, he goes on to explain how using anything for a purpose other than what it was intended will not only make the tool at least somewhat ineffective but also will usually render it worthless. Using an automobile to plow a field or a razor blade to sharpen a pencil will ruin both. Using chiropractic to get sick people well or to make chiropractors rich will similarly destroy chiropractic.

At a Philosophy Day talk at Palmer College of Chiropractic in 1992, he talked about buying a piece of material at a dry goods store. How do you know that the yard of material is truly a yard? You have a ruler or measuring device. How do we know that what we are practicing is truly chiropractic? We have a canon or measure that we use. That measure is the chiropractic philosophy.

In a 1994 lecture, he mentions one other analogy that is very important. Altering structure always affects function. When you put a suitcase on the top of your car, you have altered the structure of the car, affecting its weight, its wind resistance, its gas mileage, its braking distance, its tire wear, etc. A vertebral subluxation (change in structure) has to affect the function of the nervous system. The only thing left is to decide whether that change is bad or good.

Reggie's Quotes

1. "It's not normal to be average." - 1987

2. "Drugs don't have side effects. It's that the effects of drugs are unpredictable." - 1987

3. "You build a practice by educating patients. If you don't like talking to people, get out of chiropractic and be a cat burglar." - 1987

4. "Some people's minds are like the pupil of the eye. The more light that shines in, the more they close." - 1987

5. On the subject of changing to a family maintenance practice, "If you want to make the conversion, make the commitment." - 1987

6. "We got into chiropractic to change the world. Instead we have allowed the world to change us." - 1994

7. "A chiropractic adjustment always brings about positive changes. The mistake comes when we pretend to know what those changes will be." - 1991

8. "If medical doctors want to get rid of chiropractic, all they have to do is get sick people well." - 1972

9. "If ragweed pollen caused hay fever we would all have hay fever." - 1972

10. "If the germ theory of disease were correct there would be nobody left to believe it." - 1972

11. "No doctor anywhere ever cured anybody of anything." - 1972

12. "Every man, woman and child regardless of what disease he or she has or doesn't have needs a good nerve supply. Without it you haven't a hope in the world of staying healthy." - 1972

13. "Your body has 25 - 30 quadrillion cells." - 1972 (Apparently, science has changed the figure in the last twenty-five years.)

14. "In order to heal, the body needs no help, just no interference. -1970

15. "Most people think the brain is just a blob in the head, well it's not. It really is a blob on a stick." - 1972

16. "If chiropractic is nothing more than another treatment of dis-

ease then it is medicine." - 1988

17. "Chiropractic is different not because of what we think but because of how we think." - 1988

18. "Science is inadequate in studying life." - 1988

19. "If you were the only chiropractor left, would chiropractic survive." - 1988

20. "It's your principle that keeps you from being accepted by medicine, not your education." - 1988

21. "Under every circumstance you are better off with a good nerve supply." - 1988

22. "Chiropractic does not need a philosophy. It is a philosophy." -1991

23. On the chiropractic objective, "If you start a trip without knowing where you are going, how do you know when you have arrived." - 1991

24. "If the chiropractic philosophy is vitalistic, where do you come off with a technique that is mechanistic?" - 1991

25. "If chiropractors were paid for the last ninety six years to keep chiropractic a secret they couldn't have done a better job." - 1991

26. "I see people going to the chiropractor to get well and leaving their kids home to get sick." - 1986

27. "If you want to live to a good old age, first choose your grandparents wisely." - 1986

28. "You are what you eat is not true. You are what your body gets from what you eat." - 1986

29. "The reason for seeing a chiropractor is so that you won't be less than you should be due to vertebral subluxation." - 1986

30. "I know a guy who doctored himself for 17 years out of 'Readers Digest.' He finally died of a typographical error." - 1976

31. "What you eat for dinner tonight will be walking, talking flesh and blood tomorrow." - 1976

32. "Chiropractic is not meant to get sick people well." - 1970

33. On the importance of health maintenance, "They won't sell you life insurance in the ambulance, they know you're not a good risk." - 1970

34. On fever, "If you were to adjust to bring it down that would not be chiropractic. It would be the practice of physical medicine." - 1970

35. On waiting for symptoms, "There are people dropping dead today who never did it before." - 1970

36. On the need for universal chiropractic care, "I don't care whether he's got cancer, leprosy or rumpture gumpture of the trash bag." - 1970

37. "How can you possibly tell people that chiropractic (above-down) is right and medicine (outside-in) is wrong, when they look at you and can't tell the difference." - 1970

38. "If chiropractic got sick people well, there would be no need for any such thing as maintenance care." - 1976

39. "People are not resistant to new ideas as long as the new ideas fit into their old way of thinking." - 1970

40. "The milk of magnesia doesn't move the bowels, the bowels move the milk of magnesia because it is a poison." - 1970

41. "The average American thinks that health is being able to walk down the street in a 5 mph wind and not falling on his face." - 1970

42. "You've got to be a little cracked to let the light in." - 1970
43. "Disease is the hole that is left when health is taken away." -
44. "The man who lives for material gain as a goal for success, always dies a failure." - 1970
45. On accreditation, "If the price of recognition is to conform to the majority that are wrong, then I want no recognition." - 1971
46. On communication, "What you say is not important, what the person hears is." - 1975
47. "What you say will never be heard if it is drowned out by what you do." - 1975
48. "People are like cooked spaghetti. They can be pulled but not pushed." - 1975
49. "The most damaging lie is that freedom of symptoms means health." - 1975
50. "There is an innate awareness of every innate need." - 1978
51. "The brain and spinal cord don't run the body. A corpse has a brain and spinal cord." - 1988
52. "The difference between chiropractic and everything else is not what we think, it is how we think." - 1988
53. "We will accept anything that is consistent with our philosophy even though it's not part of it." - 1988

CHAPTER 9

Reggie

It is not as easy to understand Reggie, the man, as it is to understand his philosophy. The more you hear his message, the simpler and easier it is. However, the more you investigate the man, the more complex he becomes and the more enigmatic facts surface about him.

While Reggie may be a complex person, he is not a complex thinker. Many chiropractors have gone off in various directions only serving to make the chiropractic philosophy more confusing. Some seem to purposely complicate or distort the philosophy. Others may be just trying to take chiropractic in different directions. Reggie, on the other hand, is always trying to simplify the philosophy, to make chiropractic and the reason for being under care more readily understood. Irene says that even in discussions outside of chiropractic, he is always trying to bring those with whom he is speaking to the point. To him, the simple fact of chiropractic is "that every man, woman, and child in the world should be under regular chiropractic care." His life's work has been to simplify that message. Obviously, not everybody has a back problem or a medical disease so that has not been a part of the message. He has worked toward making it as simple as possible, while staying solidly based in irrefutable logic. Everybody needs chiropractic care and Reggie's goal is to make that need so clear that every single person on the planet will understand it.

The Man and his Message

Among Reggie's unique skills is his ability to take a person with no knowledge about chiropractic and in one hour make chiropractic the most logical, sensible idea they have ever heard. This is more than the result of being articulate. He actually brings people along so that they agree with everything he says enabling them to naturally conclude themselves the need for regular chiropractic care for a lifetime. They may not be able to explain it to someone else and unfortunately, someone may shatter that understanding later on but at that moment in time they have been drawn to a total commitment to lifetime care. The fact is they probably do not understand all the intricacies of chiropractic, but they understand enough at that moment to say, "I want regular chiropractic care for the rest of my life." I am sure many chiropractors get that kind of a response from some percentage of the people listening to their presentations, but Reggie does it with virtually the entire audience. That is a unique ability. Being able to reach the maximum number of people, many of whom have little or no understanding of his message to start with, and in a powerful enough way to cause them to make a commitment is the mark of Reggie. He, in one hour, can make someone a lifetime chiropractic patient even though they really understand little about chiropractic. Similarly, he can take chiropractors who have graduated from mixing schools and over the course of a weekend seminar turn their practices around. Many of them completely abandon the modalities and the mixing that they have been unitizing for years. They may not understand how to do it or have all of the chiropractic philosophy, they may not even have any office procedures consistent with their new found understanding, but they know after a few hours with Reggie, that they want to turn their practices and their lives around. No one else in the profession has evoked that kind of a response in so many people over a period of so many years.

How does Reggie prepare for a talk? He doesn't. Reggie tells of the time he spoke at a banquet where one of the other speakers was the only undefeated heavyweight boxing champion of the world, Rocky Marciano. Reg was sitting next to Marciano and to make conversation, he asked the great fighter how he prepared for a fight. Marciano replied, "I don't. When one fight is won, I just go back to training. I train continually." That is how Reggie does it. He is constantly thinking about chiropractic. On airplanes, in hotel rooms, wherever he is, he is thinking of ways to better explain and simplify the philosophy of chiropractic. When he is asked a question about chiropractic, regardless of how unusual the question, it seems that the answer is always right there on the tip of his tongue. That's because it is! He appears to have thought about that very concept during the preceding few minutes. Of course the fact that Reggie has been lecturing every week for the last thirty years helps to keep the philosophy in the forefront of his mind.

Reg does have a specific goal in mind for each of the different groups that he speaks to and he always gives his talk with that objective in mind. For lay people his goal is to get the children under chiropractic care. His reasoning is that children rarely have medical problems so if patients are bringing in the children, it is because they have understood what the chiropractic objective is. It is the best criteria that a patient has gotten the big idea. When speaking to chiropractic students his objective is to get them to practice and to teach the right kind of chiropractic. The objective is almost the same with chiropractors, except he has the added obstacle of trying to get them to give up some of their lucrative, nonchiropractic procedures, like modalities or insurance to practice true straight chiropractic.

To that end, Reggie is also trying to more clearly define the so-called straight mixing battle. He does not see it as a conflict between "straights" and "mixers." The lines that separate those two groups have become so muddled that the two terms are almost totally worthless. Reg wants people to understand that the difference has to do with the chiropractor's objective. If you address disease or its cause in any way, you are on one side of the fence. If you correct vertebral subluxation because it, in and of itself, inhibits an individual's ability to experience life, you are on the other side.

Reggie's message has become clearer, simpler and more focused over the years. It has also become far less vitriolic. In the early years he was the "angry young man" who fearlessly attacked medicine. Reg's antagonism toward medicine and his forensic skill were documented in a 1970 radio debate with a physician. The physician brought up the subject of vaccination and kept prodding Reg, "Do you believe in vaccinations?" Finally Reg said, "Yes I do. As a matter of fact, I would like to see every medical doctor in the United States be injected tomorrow with every vaccine they have." He went on to say, "Then while all of them are lying flat on their backs in their own hospitals, half of them dying, the public would have a chance to get well!" Through the years, the message became more focused and medicine was no longer an issue.

While Reggie is still equally strong in his philosophy, he has become less and less antagonistic toward people with other ideas. He has increasingly taken the position that chiropractic is different from anything else and everything else. Being different it does not come in conflict with anything else. As an alternative to medicine, chiropractic offends the medical doctor. As a religion, chiropractic offends people of other faiths. As a drugless healing approach, it causes a conflict with other drugless approaches as well as with medicine. By narrowing chiropractic to the simple message that Reg presents today, it does not conflict with anyone or anything else. It stands alone as a unique approach to a better expression of life by removing interference to the nervous system at the vertebral level, which can be done in concert with anything else and everything else.

Reggie readily admits that the more he has refined his message, the smaller his audience has become. The broad scope approach has always had the greater appeal in chiropractic. The more you narrow your focus, the less people are attracted to it. The irony, of course, is that the message Reg presents now has the most benefit for the most people, chiropractors and public alike. It is the way every chiropractor can have a successful, stress-free practice with no dependence upon third party pay. Yet, relatively few people are attracted to it. Similarly, with patients, Reggie's chiropractic message has benefit for every man, woman and child on the planet. If a chiropractor wanted to give a clear presentation of chiropractic to a group of people, Reggie would without doubt be the choice spokesman.

Interestingly, the market for straight chiropractic speakers is very small and limited. While Reg has spoken to hundreds and even thousands of people in past years, each weekend he can be found in some part of the country speaking to a small group of chiropractors, staff and students who are there to get nothing but chiropractic. That is Reggie's hallmark. You know you will hear nothing but chiropractic from Reg. Many of the more well-known speakers and seminars have expanded their presentations in an effort to attract a larger audience. Some, like Guy Riekman and the Quest Seminars, get into the area of personal development. Amo Bumier incorporates child birth information into his presentations and Joe Flesia has incorporated scientific and research concepts into his. This is not a criticism of them. The information they present may have great value. It simply is not chiropractic and Reggie chooses to just teach chiropractic. He acknowledges that this hurts attendance at his seminars. "I can't make a living doing seminars, there is just not that large a market... The only ones who will come are those who want my narrow viewpoint." Where other people may get one or two hundred at a seminar, Reg gets ten or twenty.

Reggie supplies his materials to the profession through a company called Chiroproducts (P.O. Box 183, Gladwyne, PA 19038, 610-649-6777). It is a source for straight chiropractic philosophy and how-to information for many straight chiropractors who would otherwise have none. Additionally, it provides follow up material for those who attend his seminars. Perhaps the most important function it serves is one that is unknown to the majority of the profession. Reg has placed video and audio tapes in chiropractic colleges libraries around the country. It is impossible to measure the influence that these tapes have had on hundreds, perhaps thousands, of students in some of the strongest mixing colleges in the country. Students who otherwise would never hear the logic of the objective straight chiropractic philosophy. Reggie also gives tapes to students. Consequently, chiropractors who purchase materials from Chiroproducts are actually helping to place Reg's message in the hands of chiropractic students around the country and the world. It also helps to defray the cost of Reggie's seminars around the country. The objective straight chiropractic message at this time appeals to so few people that Reggie cannot make a living just doing seminars alone, but very possible that will change. Chiropractic goes in cycles. One day it may very well return to the mindset of the late sixties and early seventies when there was a tremendous interest in straight chiropractic. People will be forced by increasingly thrifty insurance companies and managed care to practice the kind of chiropractic that Reggie advocates. Until that time, however, he is content to speak to small pockets of interested students and chiropractors around the country. Whatever the future holds, his tapes give us a permanent record of the man and his message.

Reggie has never written anything for commercial publication. With the exception of a few articles in various publications and of course the "Triune of Life" he has published little. Reg blames his never having written a philosophy book on his perfectionism. "I'm so much of a perfectionist that I don't want it to go out there with my name on it until it's perfect." If that is the case we may never see anything in print by Reggie because he will probably be evolving and reforming the philosophy until the day he dies. If one looks at B.J.'s writings it is easy to see a progression of thought. In later books he corrects some of the errors of earlier books. You can also see a development of the philosophy in his writings. Unfortunately, many people think a 1910 book by B.J. is just as much "gospel" as a 1945 book. This has caused quite a bit of confusion within the profession. For example, there is a group of chiropractors who practice a technique based upon a book written forty-five years ago.

It would be nice if all of the books that represented the evolving philosophy would disappear once a new edition were in print. But that does not happen. Old editions hang around and are even desired by people. This is not bad except that they are read in the context of the nineties rather than the context of the twenties or even the sixties or whenever they were written. We have all seen the damage that B.J.'s writing have done to the straight chiropractic movement, mostly because of the lack of clarity in them. It would be great if people could read B.J. in the time in which he wrote. If you understand the thinking and the philosophy of that period it helps your perspective. But even he wrote over a period of more than fifty years and he stopped writing in 1961. People who read his books and apply it to today's straight chiropractic, which has been evolving since 1961, are sometimes led astray and they distort straight chiropractic. Reg may be concerned that his books would cause the confusion that B.J.'s have. He can easily make a new tape. Anyone who has heard his audio tapes from the seventies can easily see how his philosophy has evolved. For some reason people can accept that a video or a tape made twenty years ago may become outdated, because the thinking of the speaker had changed, but when it comes to the written word, they seem to think that printed, it is unchangeable. People read B.J. as if it were canon even though early B.J. contradicts later B.J. Reg actually wrote a book on Spinology in the eighties that has never been published. A year after he wrote it, he read it and decided to rewrite it. A year later, it needed to be rewritten again. He will probably never publish a book because he constantly changes the way he sees and says things. Somehow books do not lend themselves to change. Very few people will read a book and immediately check the copyright date to see when it was published. A book is looked upon as the final word and Reggie has yet to speak his final word in chiropractic philosophy. Irene has one more reason why the man who has developed the philosophy and talked about the philosophy more than anyone else in the last three decades has not written more. She says he doesn't have the patience to sit and write. He would rather be out talking to people or thinking through the philosophy.

Reg continues to perfect the philosophy. Obviously, it is impossible to say how much further he will take it in his lifetime. There may be quantum leaps as there were with his ideas of maintenance care and non-therapeutic care, or there may simply be the fine tuning of what is now being taught. Whatever the case may be, Reg is sure to continue to develop the philosophy. Oddly enough, new insights do not seem like any major revelation to Reggie. They are more the natural progression and evolution of the chiropractic philosophy. To others, especially chiropractors or chiropractic students, his insights are often the most revolutionary ideas that they have ever heard in chiropractic. Many a student or even a chiropractor who has been practicing a long time has been blown away with the simple and logical but life-and practice-changing concepts that Reg presents. To someone who has only understood chiropractic as a treatment for back pain, the idea of regular care for every human being for a lifetime and adjusting to keep the nervous system free of interference so the individual can reach his or her full potential in life, is a monumental leap. It opens up a whole new exciting world to them and gives them a purpose that is so much more than what they had expected their lives to be.

The uniqueness of Reggie's development of the philosophy is that no matter how many changes he makes, it is still recognizable as chiropractic. If B.J. and D.D. would come back today, they would in all likelihood be in 100% agreement with where Reg has taken the philosophy. It would be nice if the same thing could be said about others in the chiropractic profession. We have seen a number of straight chiropractors who have changed the philosophy, moving either in the direction of religion or in the direction of medicine. Reg has had the unique ability to expand chiropractic while keeping it chiropractic. Very few in the history of chiropractic have been able to do that. Reg travels perhaps more than any other chiropractor in the world, including foreign countries where he lectures extensively. It might seem as if he has a mission to convert the world to chiropractic. That is really not the case. The younger Reggie was out to do this, exemplified by his now famous quote, "If you're not out to change the world, everything else is just Mickey Mouse." The older Reggie is not trying to change the world, but he is trying to change some of the people in it, or more correctly, enable them to change themselves. His message has not weakened, his zeal has not lessened but he sums it up in explaining his travel to foreign countries. "I go there for the express purpose of turning chiropractic perception around to where I think it should be. I want to get people to just look at this other viewpoint. There are a certain number of intelligent chiropractors out there and if we get them to just look at it, some of them are going to say 'Hey, that makes sense.'" That really is Reg's purpose no matter where he goes, here or abroad. To change the thinking of that percentage who are intelligent enough to see the simple message of objective straight chiropractic and to encourage them to change their practices. Regardless of how large the percentage or where they reside, Reg is going to go out and attract them with his message. He has taken his message to Australia, Japan, New Zealand, Hong Kong, England, France, Denmark, Peru, the Philippines, South Africa, Namibia, Mexico, and Puerto Rico and, of course, throughout the US.

Reggie has found that people around the world are as receptive to chiropractic as those in the United States and Canada, perhaps even more so. When he spoke to the Quechua Indians in the Andes of Peru he had to speak through two interpreters, one from English to Spanish and another from Spanish to the Indian dialect. Reg found that these Indians, who had never even seen a toaster, were receptive to the idea of regularly having their spines checked. Rarely are people in these countries as medically oriented as those in the US nor do they have a distorted idea of what chiropractic is. They do not run to a doctor or take medicine for every symptom. People who are medically oriented, including those in the US and other industrialized countries, just naturally try to fit the chiropractic doctor into that mold. Unfortunately, most chiropractors in these countries do not try to change that perception of chiropractic. They go along with it and end up treating disease. As bad as it is in this country, Reg feels that the perception of chiropractic is even worse in other industrialized countries. This country and perhaps New Zealand have the greatest percentage of objective straight chiropractors. The percentage is almost negligible in the rest of the world. That is not to say that there are not a good percentage of hands-only, spine-only chiropractors in these countries but they are treating disease.

The Man

You may get different impressions of Reggie in a social setting, depending on with whom you talk. To some, he seems somewhat shy in a crowd, almost introverted, at least compared to the articulate, gregarious person who can stand up in front of a group and talk about chiropractic for hours on end. Reggie himself, admits to being somewhat of a loner, which has perhaps developed from traveling hundreds of thousands of miles around the world by himself both as an antique buyer and a chiropractic lecturer. Reggie enjoys being in the spotlight but when the lecture or the presentation is over, he would prefer to be by himself or with a few select friends. This is not uncommon among people in the limelight. Some people have mistaken this characteristic in Reg for aloofness. They cannot understand why after speaking for five or six hours, he does not want to go to a bar with a few guys for a drink or two. They cannot understand how after doing an eight or twelve hour seminar, including answering questions before a group, he does not want to sit one on one and answer more questions. Often people do not realize how draining it is for Reg to get up in front of a group and speak. Perhaps it is because he always looks so at ease when he talks and because he always has a command of his subject matter that he appears to be completely comfortable speaking, never using notes as if he was carrying on a casual conversation with a few friends. Yet he puts tremendous energy into any talk he gives and it is draining, just as it would be for any singer or actor who may be singing a song for the hundredth time or reciting lines for a play he has been doing for six months. The mark of a great speaker or actor or singer is making it look easy. But it is not. It is hard work for any speaker, and Reg is no exception.

Reggie has a very small circle of close friends. Surprisingly, one of his closest friend is not a chiropractor. Bryan Amaral first met Reggie when Reg walked into his upscale clothing store in the Philadelphia area in 1988. The two immediately hit it off over their common interest in fine clothing. Since then Bryan has begun a business related to the garment industry and has relocated to the Atlanta area. Interestingly, when they first met Bryan was selling a very traditional line of clothing and as almost anyone knows, Reg has been anything but traditional in his clothing styles. Reg visits him in Atlanta on a regular basis and their paths often cross in other cities inasmuch as both men travel extensively. For the last two years, Reg has been trying to teach Bryan the game of racquetball, although Bryan admits Reg has not had a good deal of success in that effort. Bryan's time to devote to the game is limited, and knee injuries as an Olympic ice skater hamper the development of his racquetball skills.

Reg began to expand Bryan's vision regarding the garment industry and encouraged him to try a very entrepreneurial endeavor. Bryan has developed sophisticated computer software for the garment industry. With Reg's advice and mentoring Bryan has built a successful business. Reggie also shared chiropractic with Bryan, although very subtlety by talking about it and giving him some of his audio tapes. In addition to the friendship that has developed between the two men, Bryan is somebody with whom Reggie can discuss philosophy, life, politics and many other issues without feeling like he has to bring it back to chiropractic. Oddly enough, it is when you are discussing issues of philosophy and life unrelated to chiropractic that you often broaden your thinking and your horizons relative to chiropractic. This relationship with Bryan Amaral may do just that for Reggie. It has been a good experience for both, for Bryan because he is exposed to the philosophy of life and shares the wisdom of Reggie Gold and for Reg because he has the opportunity to discuss life with a non-chiropractor.

Thom Gelardi has created a home for Reggie in Sherman College and Reg has shown his gratitude for that by his generosity toward the College. Sherman College's Lyceum is a place for Reggie to come to every May, to rub shoulders with former students, friends and fellow straight chiropractors. While there are dozens of activities at each Lyceum, Reggie is always the main attraction, he holds center stage. Oddly enough, very few straight chiropractors have or take the opportunity to hear Reggie during the course of the year other than at Lyceum. Reg and Sherman have a symbiotic relationship. He is viewed as the "Dean of Chiropractic Philosophy," philosophy being the main emphasis of Sherman Lyceum. There is no one else in the straight chiropractic community that can move an audience to rededicating themselves to the straight chiropractic mission, to give more than they thought they had both financially and in time and effort. There is no one that can inspire an audience like Reg. All of those are a part of Sherman College's Lyceum. So the event is a benefit to both Reggie and the school. He has the opportunity to speak to his largest audience during the year. He receives the honor and respect he has earned and desires from his colleagues, the same desire he had in the Highland Regiment of the British Army. Sherman gets the most noted, most admired figure in straight chiropractic to draw a crowd and to support its mission. The present relationship between Reg and Sherman is an out-growth of the twenty-five year relationship between the school's founder and Reggie. Thom and Reggie have been through a good deal of adversity together. That adversity and the feelings between the two men have caused Reggie to consider Thom his best friend in Chiropractic.

Character Traits

One of Reggie's traits which has helped make him the force that he has been in chiropractic for over thirty years (and admittedly has also gotten him in some trouble) is his "inability to be pushed" as he describes it. He is so strong and inflexible when it comes to chiropractic and how it is practiced that often that inflexibility spills over into other areas of his life. Part of that is because chiropractic occupies so much of his life that he does not make distinctions between those areas that are not open to compromise and those areas where one can be flexible. This occurred at ADIO over the issue of whether the faculty should be paid. It was also evident in the incident that caused Reg's separation from D.E. when he could no longer accept other speakers lecturing on non-straight and anti-straight chiropractic subjects. Once, while speaking before an Australian Parliament committee on the licensing of chiropractors, Reg became very frustrated with one member of the committee who was blatantly antichiropractic. Reg finally said in frustration, "If you are going to ask and *answer* the questions, there is really no reason for me to be here." With that he got up and walked out of the hearing. A member of Parliament followed him out the door and persuaded him to return and the antichiropractic member of the committee toned down his attacks. Reg has never been much for the give and take and wheeling and dealing that is evident in politics. It is either his way or you part company, unless he can be shown that his way is not the best. Intellectually, Reg recognizes this character trait and accepts that people have differences of opinions and he does not have animosity toward people with another viewpoint. He tends to be forgiving of personal differences. He will not overlook them if he believes they are important, but he does not harbor ill-feelings toward those from whom he breaks over a difference of opinion. I recall that as emotional and traumatic as Reggie's leaving of ADIO was, he was still willing to sit down with me in a diner and objectively discuss matters that he felt were important in making the transition from his administration to the new one. Further, while we had no communication for the next five years, when our paths finally crossed at a Living Principles Seminar, Reg graciously embraced me, letting me know that even though we had had a major difference of opinion, there were no hard feelings and he welcomed a renewal of our friendship.

Reggie also has no inhibitions, which enables him to have the impact that he does. As one former student said, "He goes at everything he does with blinders on." Nothing holds him back. If something is not relative to the chiropractic philosophy, it is not worth entreating a thought of it. If it can in any way help straight chiropractic or help him help straight chiropractic, he will go after it. He is unstoppable and indefatigable in his efforts to promote straight chiropractic. Nothing and no one can stop him and plenty of people have tried in plenty of ways. He does not allow criticism or personal attacks to in any way slow him down, nor is he reticent about being in the limelight, knowing full well he will suffer attack. Reg has made mistakes, like all of us, more than he would care to admit. But he has never let a mistake keep him from his mission or even slow him down. He moves straight ahead all the time. He picks himself up and just keeps on keeping on.

Reggie is a resolver. He likes to resolve conflicts or situations even if the resolution includes walking away from it like he did with ADIO. He does not like perceived or real offenses to linger. He would rather sit down with the individual and talk it out and come to a resolution, even if that resolution meant failing to agree and parting company amiably. However, this approach often does not work for him. Reg can be very persuasive. He always argues from a position of logic, something the chiropractic philosophy has given him. And, of course, his speaking ability often makes his logic seems better than someone else's. Consequently, people are intimidated by him and often do not like to get into a one-on-one discussion or confrontation with him. They know that he may convince them that his position is correct regardless of the strength of their argument. He is such an excellent debater, having debated countless medical doctors and mixers, that one is convinced, even if he were wrong, he might still convince you to take his position. Many people are afraid to be put in that situation so they avoid him. I believe that Reg has had many strained relationships over the years because individuals were afraid to come to him and deal face to face on a particular issue.

Reggie has a phenomenal but selective memory. He does not seem to feel that keeping exact dates in his mind is terribly important. Living his life a day at a time does not necessitate that he chronicle events. Consequently, if you ask him the date of something or when a certain event took place, he is apt to give you the wrong date, not believing that time is that important. If it is of importance, he will usually say, "You'll have to ask Irene, she's good on dates." And he is right. Irene is like a walking calendar. She seems to be able to remember the date of everything.

Reg admits that he was never a very good administrator. He is too autocratic and unwilling to compromise. Unfortunately, he was forced into those situations, as in the case of ADIO, simply because the straight movement needed another chiropractic college and there was no one around to do it besides Reg. From the time Sherman was rejected by the CCE (and subsequently rejected CCE itself), the straight chiropractic leadership knew another college had to be started. It was almost three years before Reg stepped into the forefront to do it. I would venture to say had he not agreed to start ADIO in 1977, the school would have never begun. While not an administrator, Reg views himself as a pathfinder, someone who moves out in front, where no one has gone and hacks a path through the jungle. When the path is cleared and the builders come along to pave roads and put up buildings, he moves on to another jungle. So ADIO was uncharted territory and it presented a challenge to him. Perhaps that is another reason why he was willing to leave ADIO. It was in good hands philosophically and he had left it financially solvent, so he was ready to explore new territory. He wanted the chance to develop the philosophy completely apart from the idea of health, from the doctor trappings and from the encumbrances of the medical education that go along with a chiropractic education. Of course, that territory was Spinology and it took Reg and straight chiropractic to a new level.

Some have suggested that Reggie is ego driven. It seems that any strong personality is at one time or another accused of that character flaw and for some it may be true. But Reg speaks the same message to ten or fifteen people at one of his weekend seminars as he did to five hundred at the D.E. meetings of the early seventies. With a slight alteration of his message and by playing more to people's emotion he could probably attract more people or be given the opportunity to speak to more people and larger groups. But that is not important to Reg and I do not believe it ever was. He is not willing to compromise his message for an audience and if he were ego driven, he would be. Had he toned down his opposition to mixing, he might still be a speaker to the large D.E. audiences. There are a dozen or more well-known chiropractic speakers who have done just that, watered down the message for the sake of acceptance. Reggie has not and will not. It is not important to him that he stir five hundred people. It is important only that he make a difference in the life of even one person and then know that that one person will go out and make a difference in the life of just one other person. That is enough for him. That is more than most people make in an entire lifetime. Making a difference is what it is about for Reg. For others it is approbation, a large audience, the opportunity to go out and speak to a group every weekend or headline well-known seminars. They may do this but are they really making a difference in even one life? Reggie Gold is. I can personally testify to that fact. It is very much like making an adjustment. The idea is not to cure the cancer or the common cold. The idea is to make a difference. That difference may not show up in the patient for years. It may not show up for generations to come. It may not ever be noticeable. However, the adjustment is not given to make a *noticeable* difference, just to make a difference. Why do we do it? Because it is the right thing to do. That is why Reg delivers his message the way he does, with no compromise, because it is the right thing to do.

When asked what Reg's strongest point is as far as his impact upon the chiropractic profession, almost everyone associated with him is in agreement. It is his thorough knowledge of the history of chiropractic and his ability to see present circumstances in light of that history. Those that do not learn from history are doomed to repeat it and unfortunately, many in our profession have learned nothing from history. So while there may be people more knowledgeable with regard to chiropractic history, very few can see the trends of history and how they have affected and continue to affect our profession as well as Reggie Gold.

He has seen the trend toward incorporating medical practice into chiropractic to the point that chiropractic will be lost and he has fought that trend harder than anyone, including abandoning both the title of doctor and relating chiropractic to medical conditions in any way. To Reg chiropractic is one thing and one thing only. To add anything to chiropractic makes it no longer chiropractic. To take away anything from chiropractic, like its philosophy or the adjustment of vertebral subluxation, likewise makes it no longer chiropractic. That mindset is always with him and that is part of what makes him so focused in his life. He simply will not depart the chiropractic objective. He is probably one of the most singularly focused people in this world. There are many other great people in chiropractic but they have focuses other than chiropractic. Invariably, these things take them afield in chiropractic. Reg does not. Sid Williams has his love for sports and building sports complexes. Jim Parker has his desire to make people financially successful. Joe Flesia has his interest in the science of the vertebral subluxation complex. Guy Riekman is also involved in personal development. Reggie Gold will not be drawn away from chiropractic for anything no matter how good it appears to be or actually is. The only conclusion I can draw is that Reggie knows chiropractic better than any person alive. He could easily add to chiropractic and create a tremendous following. His charisma and persuasiveness is such that very few would realize it was not chiropractic, he commands such an authoritative position. Yet he does not. Because he knows chiropractic so well he knows what it is not. Keeping chiropractic pure is more important to him than anything else-ego, position, accolades, anything.

One would think that Irene Gold's insights to Reggie would be unique and different. However, Irene maintains that the Reg Gold that everyone sees is the real Reg Gold. There is no secret side to him that only she sees. There may be characteristics and qualities that she sees and others do not but that is only because of the amount of time she spends and has spent with the man compared to everyone else. He is no different in private then in public.

Irene notes that while Reggie is a very private person, he is not shy. He can walk up to anyone and begin a conversation under any circumstance, but he rarely chooses to. He is a loner and never goes to parties. Even family gatherings are usually confined to Thanksgiving. As for his personal qualities, Irene makes no apologies for being his biggest fan. "I would not be where I am today if it were not for Reggie." He encouraged her to do lay lectures, to get up in front of people to speak, to go to chiropractic college, to become a teacher and to begin doing board preparation courses which gave rise to her present and very successful Irene Gold Associates. He is very protective of her. If anything bad happens while she is out teaching, he will not tell her during their daily phone conversations. He will only share it once she has returned home.

Other qualities that Irene is more than anxious to share about Reggie are his "incredible sense of humor" and his outstanding intellect. He has a passion for people and is a very caring person toward her and toward others. His caring for people overcomes many difficulties. She says, "Reggie never lets things get to him. He doesn't hold a grudge. He has a commitment to what he is doing, he is focused so he does not let things distract him." Reg takes tremendous pride in a job well done, he is always striving to make his presentation better and, according to Irene, better is simpler. She believes his greatest contribution is "the ability to take the complex and make it simple." Irene says that his ability to use analogies, to take everyday things and relate it to chiropractic is what sets him apart. "Look at all the practice-building people and practice management consultants. They are all saying the things that he has already said."

Irene feels that among Reggie's faults is that he is too easily taken advantage of, although he does not see it that way. He maintains that it is always his choice. It is not as if he is naive. He goes into a situation fully knowing the ramifications. Why does he do it? Irene states unequivocally, "Reg knows where he is going and the legacy he wants to leave behind, which is enabling the body to reach all it can."

He is also as she puts it "not an organizational person." Reg has his own agenda and organization. You are not going to find many people who think the way he does or want to do things the way he wants to do them. He is not a

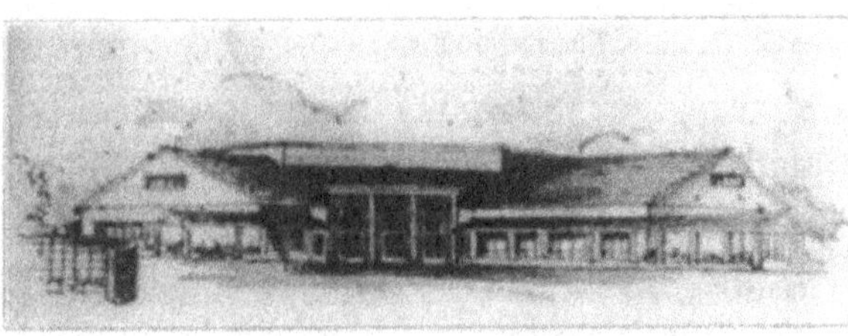

The Reginald R. Gold Building at Sherman College of Straight Chiropractic

team member, he is a leader.

From Irene's perspective Reggie's greatest honor has been the recent decision of Sherman College to name a building after him. It is indicative of his love for the school and its love for him.

Mentors

Many wonder who influenced Reggie. Who were his mentors as he learned the philosophy and grew in chiropractic? And who, if anyone, influences Reggie today? Of course, B.J. had to have been his greatest mentor. Reg went to Palmer when B.J.'s aura still very much pervaded the institution. It was not long, however, before B.J. fell out of favor even at Palmer, as he had already done in much of the profession. But while B.J. was a great influence, Reg also saw the insights and wisdom of D.D., something much of our profession has still not done. It did not lessen his respect for B.J., but Reggie saw that D.D. had some profound thoughts and had the vision of what chiropractic could be, perhaps even as much as B.J. Much of B.J.'s vision was based upon what his father had given to him.

Reg sat under the teaching of Galen Price who surely must be considered one of his earliest mentors. Reg admits he was deeply moved by the beauty and the simplicity of Price's presentation of chiropractic. It may have been that, more than anything else, that motivated him to pursue the mission of making the chiropractic message more simple, more beautiful and irrefutable to any intelligent person. To this day, Reg cannot understand how classmates of his were able to sit with him day after day and hear Galen Price explain the chiropractic philosophy and then go out and practice something other than pure, straight chiropractic. But they did.

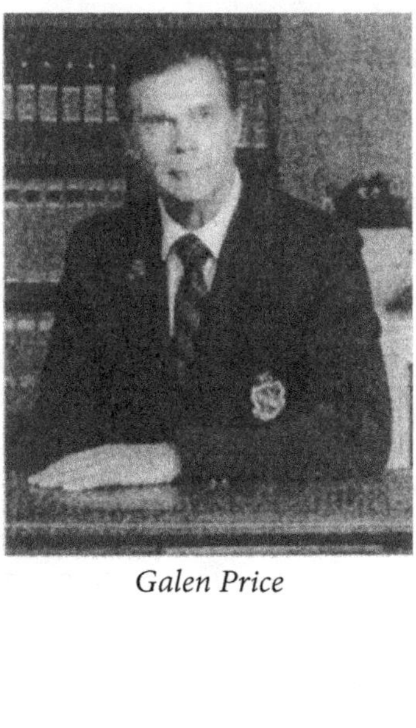

Galen Price

By Reg's definition, a mentor is not

so much someone who taught him information, but someone who taught him to think. Price taught him a deductive approach to thinking that he has applied to all aspects of his chiropractic philosophy. However, Reg notes a much earlier influence, a grade-school teacher of his by the name of Patrick Daniel Lawler. This soft-spoken, elderly Irishman taught English and literature to Reg as well as the ability to think and appreciate others' thoughts. Most of the students in the class did not respond to the man's gentle manner and genuine love for the English language, but he somehow struck a chord in young Reggie. He would write essays and poetry for Lawler that were not even assigned to the class, simply because of his love for learning, thinking and expressing thoughts. Reg credits Lawler for having instilled and drawn out these qualities in him as a young student and as such, he had deeply influenced Reg's thinking and desire to think.

After graduation, Reg went into practice and met a chiropractor by the name of Bill Bahan. Bill was one of the well-known Bahan brothers from Derry, New Hampshire who had made famous the GPC practice (box on the wall) that was begun by their uncle George Shears. Bill was very much into the chiropractic philosophy and spent many hours teaching and stimulating the thinking of the new practitioner in Spring Valley. Bahan, unfortunately for chiropractic, took his thinking out of the chiropractic realm and into the arena of religion. He formed a religion called Ontology which was based on some philosophical concepts that chiropractic embraced. Reg, of course, was able to see where chiropractic began and ended and did not follow Bahan, but he was greatly influenced by his knowledge of the philosophy. Also, through Bahan, Reg was introduced to a number of other chiropractors, a small, tightly knit group who became mentors for each other. Dan McGauren from Nyack, New York was one of this group. He had actually been the one who had introduced Reggie to Bahan. Dan was another strongly principled, philosophically sound chiropractor who, despite his soft-spoken and quiet manner, had an unquestionable love and zeal for straight chiropractic.

There have been many others. No single person has ever been

"The Mentor" to Reg. There are dozens of chiropractors that have influenced him, each of whom has opened small windows of understanding in his development. He honestly considers his students to be his greatest mentors, in the sense that they, more than anyone, have stimulated him to think. No one asks questions like a student and a teacher feels more obligated to answer the questions of students. I personally have labored over students' questions to make sure that the next day I had an answer. One might tend to shrug off a chiropractor's question, but feel compelled to think through an answer for a student. This, more than anything, stimulated Reg's thinking. What is more, being the undisputed expert in chiropractic philosophy, he has probably had his thinking stimulated in this manner more than any other chiropractic teacher, primarily because he has been asked more and tougher questions than anyone over the years. He has, no doubt, had hundreds of students try to play "stump the professor." That is not to suggest that all the questions ever asked of Reg were done in an adversarial manner. Many were asked simply because the student was encouraged to think. Questions are a result of someone thinking and no one can cause an individual to think and critically evaluate their present thinking more than Reggie Gold. Of course, those students in turn challenged him and his philosophy, causing him to think and develop that philosophy. This give and take relationship between him and his students has been an important part of his life, his teaching and his own philosophical development. As he looks back today, he realizes he was totally unprepared to teach philosophy at Columbia (of course, there was no one else any better prepared) but he learned from the students' challenge. That was a unique aspect of his learning experience.

When he went to Sherman he met a different group of students with a different mindset and of course, different questions. By this time he was teaching a different model of chiropractic, so it was expected that a new set of questions would be elicited. Today, he is meeting a third type of student, one that is very scientifically oriented. Reggie's challenge is to find answers to their questions that are simple and logical and that can refute the pseudoscientific mindset that is forced upon them. Much of what purports to be science is totally illogical and science must conform to the laws of logic. Reggie's effort has been making straight chiropractic logical to the student and demonstrating the absurdity and illogic of much of what is being taught. Whether he is speaking before a group of students at Sherman or at Western States is irrelevant. The message is the same, simple and logical. As far as Reg is concerned, if you are logical, you must accept chiropractic. Reg admits that much of the learning he has done, that has enabled him to answer questions, has come from outside of chiropractic in diverse areas such as Socratic philosophy and religion. Reg has been influenced by Plato's *Republic* and the writings of Ayn Rand. The Greek mythological story of Sisyphus, King of Corinth, has also greatly affected Reggie and influenced his thinking. Sisyphus one day saw an eagle, greater than any mortal one, carrying off a maiden to a nearby island. Later the river god Asopus told him that his daughter, Aegina, had been abducted and Asopus suspected Zeus. He asked Sisyphus if he would help him find Aegina. Sisyphus related what he had seen and as a result he incurred the wrath of Zeus. His punishment was to be in Hades forever, where he would have to push a rock up a hill. Just before he got to the top, the rock would roll back down and he was forced to start over. Sisyphus won in the end, however, for he did not take his joy from the accomplishment, the completion of the task which would forever elude him. He took his pleasure from the effort.

Throughout his lifetime in chiropractic, Reggie has had to push many rocks uphill only to have them roll back down the hill. Some of them have been due to his own decisions like leaving a successful practice, the top practice in the world at the time, to become a teacher in a new chiropractic college. Some of the rocks have been totally outside of his control. But each time he has begun again. Reg does not seem to be discouraged by anything. His joy is in the struggle, in pushing the rock up the hill. Reg does not let negatives deter him. If the joy is in the pushing, it doesn't matter if the rock rolls back down the hill and you have to start again. He just does not let adversity bother him. Either he ignores it as he did with the negative response of much of the profession toward Spinology or he walks away from it. If he walks away, he does not dwell on the incident or let it fester. He forgets it and moves on. This ability to avoid hypersensitivity is an important trait for any successful person to have. Reg does not let rejection defeat him. If it does bother him somewhat, it does not deter him from his task. If he concerned himself with how the profession would react to Spinology, he would have never started it. If he worried about how the profession would accept his new ideas as far as the philosophy and practice of chiropractic were concerned, he never would have presented them. He does not worry that a percentage of those hearing his message are going to reject it, he focuses on the percentage that will accept it, even if that percentage is a minority.

This ability was probably developed in his practice in Spring Valley. As good as he was at communicating chiropractic, Reg estimates that only 10 - 12% of the patients got the message of regular, lifetime, family care. When as many as 90% reject your message, you must become strong and resistant to that rejection and focus on the 10% that are accepting it. Reggie was able to do that in practice and it has carried over to his teaching and his vision. The rest of the chiropractic profession has had difficulty learning that concept. Many within our profession are trying to impress the medical community so that they will stop rejecting us or stop saying bad things about us. We even spent millions of dollars as a profession to get them to stop. We sued them at a period when chiropractic had reached an unprecedented level of acceptance. Reg never cared what medicine thought or said about him. It was never worth thinking about.

Many in our profession are worried about what the patients will think about our care or inability to get them well. That is why they mix. What our profession should be doing and saying is, "Here is what I do. If you want it fine, if not I'll move on. But I can't compromise what I do or do something else so that you will accept me or think more highly of me." Reggie has grasped that idea and applied it to his life. His work is too important. He believes if he focuses on the negative he will become negative. He puts it this way, "If I'm driving my car along the road and a mad dog barks at my car, I don't get out of the car and bark back, I know where I'm going." He wants acceptance as much as the next guy but he wants acceptance of *his* idea and what *he* stands for.

Reggie is a tremendously self-confident person, in many areas. Self-confident people, however, are often perceived as being arrogant. Because of his self-confidence and lack of confidence in many others, Reggie has taken upon himself the dominant role in movements and organizations. He took some of these roles simply because he believed himself to be the best person to do the job, others because nobody else wanted them. This is not arrogance, it is self-confidence. Every chiropractor who accepts a patient has this confidence otherwise he or she would logically refer the person to another chiropractor. So it is normal to have confidence. Anything less would be a false humility. Great things are not accomplished in this world by people who have a self-deprecating attitude. Reggie has no such attitude. He is the best communicator and the best visionary thinker in straight chiropractic. But when he speaks, he does not present his ideas in an arrogant way. He does not expect that what he says will be accepted because of who he is. He expects that his message will be accepted because it is simple, logical and strikes a chord in the listener's thinking. That is not the presentation of an arrogant person. He has an authoritative air about him. He has a certain charisma about him. But those are not the things that impress you when Reggie Gold speaks. It is never the man; it is always the message. If you reread the accolades in the front of this book, the emphasis is invariably on how Reggie has changed the individual's thinking or his or her vision or way of looking at chiropractic. In discussing this book, he wanted to be sure that even the title reflected the message, not only the man. In a profession sorely lacking sound leadership, this is just the type of person needed. Even before B.J.'s death, the profession had no one to step up as a leader, at least not in the straight chiropractic community. Dave Palmer was simply incapable of doing the job. It is obvious, during that period, that no one assumed the mantle of B.J., for it was at this time that the mixing aspect of the profession took control of the national association and the accrediting agency and became the spokesperson for the chiropractic profession in general.

Reggie rose to the top of the straight chiropractic community at just the right time. It was not so much that there was a lack of political leaders, administrators, competent chiropractic college presidents or entrepreneurs, there were many of them. When it comes down to it, those are not necessarily Reggie's strong suits. What was sorely lacking was leadership in the vision of chiropractic. The profession, even the ICA was drifting farther and farther away from chiropractic. The procedures "complimentary to" the adjustment were becoming more and more important to chiropractic practice. Reggie had the foresight not to try to stop the drift of straight chiropractic toward mixing, but to move it in an entirely new direction. It is clear, both from history and from looking at the present status of the traditional straight chiropractic community, that the profession could not stay where it was, correcting vertebral subluxations to get sick people well. It had to either move in a direction focusing less and less on disease and more and more on human potential or else be assimilated by therapeutic chiropractic. If Reggie had tried to maintain the status quo, even that of B.J.'s chiropractic, chiropractic may have disappeared entirely. The actions and philosophy of those traditional chiropractors who espouse B.J. philosophy testify to the truth in the above statement. They are focusing on getting into hospitals to treat back problems. They are into diagnosis, sports medicine, nutrition and most of all, while they give lip service to an innate philosophy, their practice hardly aligns with the principles of removing interference to the expression of the body's innate wisdom and then stepping back. Moving chiropractic away from medicine and toward the original ideas of B.J., innate expression, is the visionary leadership that Reg has given to the chiropractic profession.

Other Interests

Reggie has a wide variety of interests, however, only his closest friends ever get a glimpse at them. It is almost as if he fears that should people perceive other things in his life besides chiropractic, it will somehow lessen their ardor, dedication and commitment to perpetuating straight chiropractic. Even the most dedicated of chiropractors need little encouragement to allow other things to get into their lives and distract them from their chiropractic mission. Consequently, you will rarely hear Reggie publicly discuss any of his outside interests, with one major exception. For many years, wherever he went to speak, he would always look for some racquetball competition. He might even announce from the platform that he would enjoy a game of racquetball and he would often travel to a speaking engagement a day early just to play racquetball with a local chiropractor. He would purport to be looking for the exercise that a friendly game of racquetball would give him. The truth is Reg enjoys every aspect of the game especially the idea of winning by beating his opponent senseless.

Reg first got interested in the game in the seventies when he came to Pennsylvania to begin ADIO, about the same time the game was becoming popular. One of the students at the school worked in a racquetball club and one evening Reg was able to rent the entire club for the students, faculty and administration. He had never played the game but was hooked after that first night. It helped keep him in physical shape and enabled him to get rid of some of the frustration of trying to run the school. Many a young chiropractor has been surprised and shocked at not only Reg's ability to play the game but also his fierce competitiveness. Reg has a desire to succeed at whatever he does and the game of racquetball is no exception.

Although he does not actively participate in other sports, Reggie does have an interest in watching them and is capable of conversing on an intelligent level about football. He has taken to the Philadelphia sports teams and has been known to discuss the finer points of the game in front of the television. Reg also enjoys watching golf on television. Once after being together at a seminar where we both lectured, I asked him what his plans were for the remainder of the day. I was getting ready to leave for the airport and he seemed to be in no particular hurry. He said he was going back to his hotel room to watch a golf match he was particularly interested in seeing. As a non-golfer, I find the idea of watching it on television to be terribly boring, Reg does not.

Some of his interest lies in understanding the strategy of the game or the sport, whether it is a high contact sport like football, like golf, or like a good game of chess. Reg was founder of the Chess Club at Palmer College back in his student days. All necessitate strategy and I'm sure Reggie's interest in understanding the strategy of sports helps him in chiropractic. Some of the greatest strategists in football, for example outstanding coaches, have never even played the game or were merely ordinary players. Further, the wisdom of a Vince Lombardi or a John Wooden is often used by motivational people and those involved in impacting peoples' lives. A lot can be learned from these people and applied to the game of life and chiropractic. Reggie has been in enough chiropractic battles and chiropractic wars to appreciate the need for strategy. Further, every day we as chiropractors are in a war, a battle for the minds of human beings, getting them to understand our above-down philosophy over and against the outside-in philosophy. Any principles of strategy that can help in that regard are worthwhile. Of course, there is always the possibility that Reg just enjoys the game. One thing is for sure, Reg never develops a passing interest in anything. If he wants to know about something like football, he wants to know all about it. If he learns to play racquetball, it is not for exercise, fun or fellowship with another chiropractor. It is for keeps. He wants to beat every opponent who steps on the court with him.

Dick Plummer is one of the few people who is able to converse with Reg about subjects other than chiropractic. In fact, Dick and his wife Joann, have traveled to England with Reg and Irene simply for the fun of a vacation. Dick recalls one occasion when a young chiropractor found out that he had had Reggie to his house. The chiropractor was eager to know what they had talked about in such a setting. Dick explained that they had discussed, among other things, can openers. The chiropractor was curious as to what esoteric concepts the can opener could hold as to warrant discussion by the world's most notable chiropractic philosopher. Dick had to explain that these were no deep metaphysical concepts. Reggie and he both do a good deal of cooking and they were simply discussing how hard it is to find a dependable can opener. One might think it strange to picture Reggie Gold in the kitchen, but considering the amount of time he spends eating in restaurants and the busy schedule that Irene keeps with her Review courses, it is understandable that he would take an interest in cooking if for no other reason than survival.

Anyone who has been in Reg's home can see that he has more than a passing interest in art. He seems to appreciate all kinds of art and his walls and living room are full of everything from beautiful paintings to primitive African wood carvings. He had for many years a stuffed elephant's leg as an end table! The design of his home, with its high ceilings, creates a wall almost thirty feet high and twenty feet wide as you enter the foyer. It is covered with nothing but paintings to the ceiling, many of which are collector's items. While objects of art are a hobby and of interest to him, they do occupy a proper place in the scheme of things. It perhaps goes back to his days in the antique business and why he left it. While they do add an appreciation for beauty and the human spirit to people's lives, as mentioned previously, Reg says that if another antique was never bought or sold, humanity would be little the worse for it. That thinking motivated him to leave the antique business and get into chiropractic and that understanding of life's priorities has not changed.

Reggie also enjoys talking politics. One might guess that he is rather liberal in his politics but the truth is quite the contrary. Those that have discussed the subject with him say he is quite conservative. In this way, he has a balanced viewpoint of life. He has a love for humanity but realizes that people are best served by allowing them to take control of their own lives, whether it is in the area of health care or in matters of their personal life. He very rarely, however, talks about subjects other than chiropractic except with a select few people. Most chiropractors, even those that have known him for years, have probably never heard his political viewpoints, his thoughts on the Philadelphia Eagles quarterback problems or his opinion on Australian wines, another subject he has made a point of becoming somewhat of an expert on because of his many trips to that country.

Reg is also something of a designer and architect. His home in Gladwyn, Pennsylvania is an absolutely beautiful structure, much of which he designed himself. Reg is also responsible for much of the interior decor, above and beyond his exceptional art collection. The most striking aspect of the home is the way it compliments the surrounding landscape. Most homes have landscaping that is designed to compliment the house, that is, the house is the primary focus. But when you drive through the pillars and up the long path that leads to the Gold residence, you are struck by the way the home blends into the surrounding hilly and wooded landscape. The property is thick with both deciduous and evergreen trees and the home somehow looks like part of the landscape rather than something built in it or on it. Reg designed the rocky stream bed that meanders down the property and even did some of the work himself, moving rocks to give it the natural effect that he desired. There is also a natural stream at the lower end of the property. Water is pumped from there to a pond at the upper end. The pond overflows to the rocky stream bed and runs through the property eventually emptying into the stream from where it originated. The gurgling brook flows by Reg's private office and the sound can be heard through the open office windows. The landscaping is particularly beautiful in the early spring when the azaleas are in bloom. In the summer when the trees and foliage are full, you cannot see either of his two neighbors' homes. Reg, being a very private person, does not know one of his two neighbors. The other is the man who built Reggie's house. His home definitely exemplifies his philosophy of "things natural."

Anyone who has ever been to any of his homes in New York, South Carolina or Pennsylvania realizes one thing very quickly, Reg loves animals, especially dogs. Reggie has always had dogs even as a boy. Big dogs and small dogs, but mostly big dogs. He has no preference as far as breed is concerned. When he lived in Yardley, he had four of them. Upon entering the driveway leading to his present home you are first greeted by two, large, stone dogs sitting atop the pillars, guarding both sides of the entrance. After passing through the gate, which always seems to be open, you are greeted by the sudden appearance of a rather large, live dog (Reggie's Dalmatian, Domino). He will follow, even lead you to the parking area, check you out momentarily and then return to more interesting endeavors. Reg and Irene have also recently acquired Mr. Katz, a black, white and gray cat, who has since taken over the house. He has even been spotted sleeping right in the middle of Reg's personal desk.

Reg is an avid reader, reading over one hundred books a year and his tastes are as varied as one could imagine. He has read everything by Leon Uris, James Michener and Tom Clancy, three very diverse writers. If there are common threads among these writers that attracts Reggie, they include the excellence with which they develop the plot, the characters and the places as well as the highly technical aspects of their writing. There are many excellent writers but there are very few who will take the time and make the effort to develop a plot to the degree that these three do. Reggie admires that desire for perfection in others, whether in writing, playing tennis, golf or curling. He once stayed up until 3 AM on a seminar weekend in Canada watching a curling match on the hotel television. Most people probably do not even know what curling is. It is a game originating in Scotland in which two four-person teams slide heavy oblate stones toward the center of a circle at either end of a length of ice. He was intrigued by the skill they demonstrated. Reggie also enjoys reading philosophical treatises and poetry. History fascinates him, especially the War between the States. It is understandable that he would have an interest in history because most of history represents the thinking of various people. It is a perfect demonstration of the chiropractic principle of cause and effect. All of the factors, circumstances, attitudes, and philosophies of people on both sides of the Mason-Dixon line converged to become the cause of the Civil War which is still having an effect on this country today. It is interesting to see which causes came together to create the effects that occurred and to see that if even one of those causes were changed, history would be altered. It is particularly interesting to someone who talks every day about changing the world. When you look at history, it is easy to see how a small thing can change the world. It has been suggested that Napoleon's hemorrhoids affected his decision making at Waterloo. Had he been healthy, the history of western civilization might well be different than it is today. As a student of history, Reg has seen how "small things" can alter the course of history. This as well as anything causes him to see the importance of changing the thinking of even one person. When it comes to reading, Reggie is as intense about his books as he is about everything else in his life. Recently he was on a plane reading *Redemption* by Leon Uris. The book deals with the oppression of the Irish people by the English. That he could handle. After all, he has been a part of an oppressed group (i.e., chiropractors) for over thirty years. But on this particular flight home from Atlanta, he came to a part where the estranged father of the main character wrote his son a letter saying he would like to reconcile before he died. Reg was so touched by the scene that tears rolled down his cheeks.

The Generous Giver

Reggie's generosity to Sherman College of Straight Chiropractic is well known by the profession, especially since his 1994 donation of $125,000. That in addition to numerous other gifts to the school through the years, should give him a special place in the hearts of everyone even remotely associated with Sherman College.

The mark of a great giver is not what he gives out of his abundance, but what he gives out of his limited wherewithal. Contrary to what some may think and even the impression he has given Reggie has never been a wealthy man. He had a successful antique business before going to Palmer but he still had to work three jobs to get through chiropractic college. He borrowed money and depended upon the generosity of Dr. Pepper to get him started in practice. He lived in a very nice home in Spring Valley, wore nice clothes and drove an expensive car but he was far from being a rich chiropractor. You do not get rich with a box on the wall practice, even seeing 1500 or more patients a week, especially if you have associates running the practice. Being out of the office during the Spring Valley years surely hurt him financially. Often the fee or the honorarium given to travel somewhere to speak did not even cover the expenses and he never received a cent when he traveled to speak to other chiropractors' patients.

When Reg left Spring Valley to go to Sherman, he suffered a tremendous drop in income. Reggie practically gave the practice and home away, a generous gesture considering the size of the practice. Irene was still finishing education at Columbia. Much of Reggie's generosity is unseen and in reality dwarfs the 1994 gift to Sherman although that has gotten the most publicity. Reggie really does not like the limelight as far as his generosity is concerned. The Sherman article regarding the donation that appeared in various professional publications was more for Sherman's benefit. The college was going through a difficult period because of their lack of accreditation and was working toward being accredited by CCE. It needed the profession and the accrediting agency to see that it had donors who were willing to give substantial sums of money to support the college. Reg is anxious to give. He wants to be generous in life rather than death, so that he can see the fruits of his giving. He points to Anton Meister, another great New York chiropractor from Palmer who left great sums to his alma mater only to have it eaten away to relatively little by lawyers and probate. Reg is giving his legacy away during his lifetime.

His generosity does not extend only to recent times. On one occasion when PACE was doing a fund raising and raffling off an automobile, the raffle went particularly badly for some reason. Rather than let it lose money, Reggie put a couple thousand dollars of his own money into the raffle to make it a success on the books. Other stories concerning Reggie's generosity abound. As one of the sponsors of the P.A.C.E. Testimonial and Farewell Dinner honoring Reggie held in Liberty, NY in August of 1973, Thom Gelardi writes: "Best wishes to Dr. Reginald R. Gold who gives and gives and gives." Thom recognized Reggie's generosity even in his early association with him. Reggie is not interested in sharing other stories of his generosity, so much of it will continue to go unnoticed.

Slings and Arrows

Reggie has been the target of attacks by many people over the years. Obviously, by taking a strong, non-compromising position, he put himself in line for attack. Reg has no problem with professional attacks from those that might attack his philosophy or his position on an issue. He expects that, it comes with the territory. He, in fact, welcomes that type of controversy. As B.J. said in the title of one of his later books *Conflicts Clarify.* The conflicts that Reggie has been involved in (and sometimes created) have helped to clarify straight chiropractic. He considers it to be a privilege to be criticized for speaking the truth. Those attacks make him stronger, convince him of the importance of his message and his work. Unfortunately, Irene has not handled those attacks on Reg as well. It is especially hard on her when she sees people who Reg has helped tremendously to build a practice turn on him. On more than one occasion she has suggested to Reggie that he get out of chiropractic, that the profession is not worthy of his efforts and time. Irene is probably right, but Reggie doesn't do what he does for the profession, he does it for humanity. In one of his recent tapes he says that he does not care about helping chiropractors build large successful practices, he cares about getting the world under regular chiropractic care and that is what he is helping chiropractors to do. Irene says that his response to why he puts himself in such situations where people attack him was "that if he couldn't stand the heat he should get out of the kitchen." Reggie Gold has stood a great deal of heat in his chiropractic lifetime and Irene has always taken things harder than

Reg. A recent example of the attacks that indicate he is stirring up the profession was the purposeful exclusion of him from the video produced for the 100th year celebration produced by Guy Riekman and the Centennial Committee. Riekman actually decided to quit over Reggie's exclusion, but Reggie convinced him to stay with the project. As an important figure in the history and development of the chiropractic profession, Reggie clearly deserved to be a part of the video. In fact, he was interviewed and included in an earlier version of it. The fact is that much of the earlier portion of the final video discussed the changes in how health care is viewed, the need for a new model in health care for the coming century and the part that chiropractic plays in the human potential movement. Reg Gold, more than anyone else, is responsible for the development of that model within the chiropractic profession. In the last twenty years he has set chiropractic on that road more so than any other figure in chiropractic today. For that reason alone, he deserved, at the absolute least, an obligatory mention. Reg takes a very gracious attitude toward ending up on the cutting room floor largely because of the efforts of certain influential chiropractors (a few with thick wallets). He says that it is encouraging to know that his message is so powerful and effective that those chiropractors feared his inclusion in the video. However, I cannot help but think that Reggie also is understandably hurt that his contribution to chiropractic was not acknowledged in this supposedly important documentation of the profession's first one hundred years. Reg wants his contribution to be remembered and recognized. That is only human. The Centennial Video unjustly denied him that recognition.

The first incident in his practice that hurt personally was when he was accused of false and misleading advertising while in Spring Valley, New York. During his entire time in practice, Reggie never advertised. Not that he felt there was anything wrong with it, he encouraged it under PACE, it simply was not necessary to his practice. Besides, it was illegal. The incident related in Chapter 2 caused him considerable embarrassment because it was an attack upon his reputation and professionalism. As much as it hurt him, he felt worse for

Irene who had to deal with it while he was lecturing in South Africa.

The next personal attack was more than verbal or ludicrous charges. It was upon his physical person and property. While living in South Carolina, he raised the ire of a local chiropractor. The chiropractor, who was a deacon in his local church, announced that there were devil worshippers living at 1028 West Main Street. It is true that in the early seventies Reggie was anything but conventional and conservative. He also had Sherman students at his home constantly, some of whom were those of the sixties generation, so their appearance and demeanor was most likely a little out of the ordinary for the deep south. For example, P.J.

On a number of occasions, some of these Southerners came driving through the property firing shotguns and other weapons. One night a shotgun blast ripped through P.J. Martin's teepee. Had she been standing up rather than lying down sleeping, she most surely would have been killed. Reggie was no longer on the faculty at Sherman at this time so he was often not at home but away lecturing. Consequently, Irene was forced to live through these attacks without him. It got to the point where students from Sherman would arm themselves and come to ADIO House when Reggie was away to protect Irene. On at least one occasion, a running gun battle occurred between the students and the "drive by shooters." Again, Reggie's concern was for Irene and any student bystanders. Fortunately, before anyone was hurt, the shootings ceased. One night Reggie "got the drop" on a group of them and invited them to his home for a cookout. He showed them his extensive collection of African artwork. Apparently a witch doctors mask on the front door had contributed to the misunderstanding about "devil worship." Reg eventually got some of them under chiropractic care.

Another incident involved a well-known chiropractor from South Carolina who had tremendous influence over the South Carolina State Board. He informed Sherman that the Board would never approve the school as long as Reggie was there. The school could not continue without that approval because they needed to open the student clinic and the Board had to give approval for students to adjust even under supervision. When Thom Gelardi approached Reg with this news, Reggie resigned for the good of the school but it had to have been a very painful experience for him. A group of students rebelled against the idea of Reggie leaving and wanted to fight the state board on this issue. However, Reggie realized the college had enough battles to fight and that this one would jeopardize those very students' right to adjust in the Health Center and he personally stopped the student rebellion.

His departure from ADIO was another painful experience for Reggie. When your opposition attacks you because they do not understand or agree with you as with the South Carolina State Board or the Centennial Committee that is one thing. When total strangers attack as with the drive-by shootings that is also understandable. But the pain in the ADIO incident was that this time his opposition was his friends and allies in the school. They precipitated his decision to resign. It was not over principle or philosophy, it was over personnel policy. While Reg left the school he started in the hands of people who were philosophically straight, it was painful knowing that those who shared his vision did not have enough confidence in him to give him the freedom to develop the school as he felt best.

or philosophy, it was over personnel policy. While Reg left the school he started in the hands of people who were philosophically straight, it was painful knowing that those who shared his vision did not have enough confidence in him to give him the freedom to develop the school as he felt best.

Reggie realizes he is going to get shot at, at least verbally, because he is out front. He says, "If you don't want to be shot at stay behind with the troops. A true leader is out front." Reggie has taken so many shots and has chosen to remain out front where you receive more attacks, that people seem to think he thrives on it. Quite the opposite is true. Reggie is a very sensitive person. He is hurt by attacks upon his person. But being the private person that he is, he does not show the pain and except for a few close people, he rarely shows the fact that he is hurting. The personal injury that he suffers does make him stronger. If it involves chiropractic philosophy, he will work harder to make the philosophy simpler, easier to understand and more acceptable to more people. That is the best way he finds to answer his critics, convert more people to his way of thinking. If it is a personality conflict, he will just move out in another direction with more resolve to succeed in what he is doing. Criticism or compliment, attacks or accolades, Reggie Gold is driven by chiropractic, to serve chiropractic. He has a personal sense of destiny.

CHAPTER 10

Man On A Mission

No one can predict the future, especially that of another individual since future events are always determined by our decisions and acts of our own volition. I believe, however, it is safe to say that in one way or another Reggie will be associated with the principle of what we now call objective straight chiropractic. Reggie's involvement depends a good deal on the direction of chiropractic as a profession. Reg himself believes that the rift between objective straight chiropractic and the rest of the profession is widening. If the straight chiropractic community can hold on, and with the CCE's approval of Sherman that is looking very likely, the difference will one day be so great as to split chiropractic into two professions. One group will become medical doctors or chiropractic physicians in the true sense of physician and the other group will embrace chiropractic only. Reg believes that about 95% of the profession wants to go the medical way. Actually, he says that 50% are strongly committed to it and the other 45% will go along either because it is financially more lucrative, because it is what they have been taught or because they choose to align themselves with the majority. How long this will take is anybody's guess, but as quickly as it is moving Reg sees it conceivably occurring in the next twenty-five years. If that is the case, then we are in for an exciting period in chiropractic. I am sure Reggie will be at the forefront of the straight movement, if not physically, his spirit, his thinking and his perspective will permeate every fiber of that entity we call straight chiropractic and will have a profound effect upon its continued growth and evolution.

Reg Gold has given us more than tools for communicating or a hundred good analogies and the desire to communicate chiropractic. He has given us a way to think and a desire to think. Robin Williams best describes it in *Dead Poets Society.* Williams' character says, "Just when you think you know something, you must look at it in a different way." Reggie has constantly challenged us as chiropractors to look at chiropractic in a different way. When he first graduated from chiropractic college, the vision he shared with us was what he was taught, "chiropractic gets sick people well." He thought chiropractic could grow a new arm on a one-armed man. Perhaps, it was Reggie's own personal experience with allergies that really did not improve for many years despite regular chiropractic care, that helped develop his philosophy. When you, yourself, do not get well and even develop problems under chiropractic care and/or the same can be said about many of your good patients, it makes you think. It is at this point many chiropractors reject the philosophy and begin to mix. They overlook the simple, logical explanation that Reggie is largely responsible for giving to the chiropractic profession. His conclusion was that just maybe chiropractic is not meant to get sick people well. Not only is it not a cure-all, it is not a cure-anything. It is intended to do one thing, allow the innate intelligence of the body to be better expressed and therefore allow the individual's body to work better. Once Reggie was able to accept this concept, his practice and his approach took on a whole new and totally different dimension. It was a freeing experience.

Reg's concept of chiropractic evolved to chiropractic for a better expression of health for everyone, regardless of the body's ability to heal itself. When he had fully developed that concept and given it to chiropractors who were first talking prevention and health maintenance, he began to look at chiropractic in a different way. Increasing an individual's human potential was just another way of looking at the philosophy of straight chiropractic. The ramifications of that vision of chiropractic are enough to keep Reggie thinking for ten lifetimes, but who knows what new insights or ideas he will share with us during the remainder of his lifetime. Quoting Williams' character again, Reggie has never feared to "strike out on new ground." This is part of his legacy to the chiropractic world.

Reggie would like to be remembered as someone who simplified chiropractic, who made it attractive and understandable to every chiropractor and every lay person. He has done that but not because of his eloquent speech or dynamic presentation. It is because he has been able to touch the part of the human soul that thinks. He has reached that part of each individual that uses reason, that makes decisions and looks at life in a logical way.

Reggie came into the profession at a perfect time. The authority figure in chiropractic, B.J. Palmer, was no longer a force. The profession was dividing into two groups. The dogmatic segment of the profession was willing and anxious to form an almost cult-like organization around the teachings of B.J. They held onto all of B.J.'s writings as if they were holy scripture and considered themselves traditional straight chiropractors. The other group consisted of those that embraced the religion of scientism. They were unwilling to accept any of the philosophical concepts of chiropractic. They were mechanists in the true medical model. If chiropractic could be empirically demonstrated to relieve musculoskeletal conditions, that would be more than enough to satisfy them. Both groups hold no future for chiropractic. The first is an untenable, indefensible position that would relegate chiropractic to a small Christian Science-like following. Their "cause of all disease" philosophy would not be acceptable to an increasingly sophisticated society. The second group would at best cause chiropractors to be absorbed by medicine like the osteopath, at worst (although both seem equally bad) as a physical therapist. Reggie gave us a third view, a rational, reasonable way of looking at chiropractic. It maintains the objective of B.J.'s chiropractic and could satisfy any reasonable scientist. Reg sees his message as simple and perhaps it is, but the beauty of it is not its simplicity but its logic. Any person using their sound mind, who has a viewpoint of life that accepts a universal intelligence is forced to accept the chiropractic philosophy as Reggie Gold presents it.

When one looks closely at Reggie, it is amazing how much foresight he demonstrates. In the past few months, I have become more and more convinced that the term "doctor" and the disease-treating image that it evokes is one of the great hindrances to the profession's advancement. That was demonstrated in the mid-seventies when CCE came into power and the ICA schools began to use the excuse that since we were doctors we must diagnose. As objective straight chiropractic, we argued that point and while it is true that it does not require us to diagnose, the association of the term "doctor" with disease treatment is almost universally accepted. Reg was talking about getting rid of the term eighteen years ago, that is one reason why he began Spinology. Even when he got back into chiropractic in 1986, he still held to that position. In a letter to the editor of *Chiropractic Conversations* (Vol. 5, No. 1), he stated:

> "As you know, I left chiropractic because I felt that my idea of non-therapeutic spinal practice could not succeed when the people practicing it called themselves 'Doctor;' were licensed to practice a healing art and called the persons who visited them 'patients.' My ideas in this regard have not changed."

Reggie claims to be happier and more contented than he has ever been in his life. If appearances are any indicator, then he surely is. He no longer has the unpleasant challenges of politics and the associated negatives. His only challenges are philosophical and communication, making the philosophy as simple as possible and teaching chiropractors to effectively communicate it. There are fewer challenges. Only the ones he himself creates. Reggie has to deal with no one but himself and his seminar attendees. No state boards, no Board of Trustees, no administrators, no politicians, just himself and those who are interested in his message.

One desire that has driven him is the desire for acceptance, beginning from his early military career. At this time in history, Reg is enjoying the greatest amount of acceptance and respect for himself and his message yet. There are a number of reasons for this. First, he has simplified his chiropractic message to its most easily understood, logical and hence, acceptable form. Second, he no longer is attacking medicine or mixers and third, and most important, there is now a generation of leaders in the chiropractic profession who have been exposed to Reggie and his message. Many of them were young students who heard Reggie either on or off campus at chiropractic colleges all over the country. Reggie's willingness to go to any college and speak to any number of students for the last twenty years is now reaping results. They may not have fully accepted his approach to chiropractic but they have developed a respect and an admiration for this man who has had a passion for straight chiropractic and a desire to share it with everyone. They also know that those trips to speak to them were out of his own pocket, simply because he wanted to share a message with them. That kind of dedication commands respect. Respect for Reg can only increase because Reggie is daily impacting upon students who will be the future practitioners and leaders of the profession. His tapes are in college libraries and he presently speaks on and off college campuses about twelve to fifteen times a year.

As a side-effect of Sherman College's acceptance into the chiropractic fraternity, Reggie who has been and is still closely associated with the college has been "legitimized." This has further added to his acceptance by the chiropractic community. Some CCE schools even feel comfortable inviting him to speak to the students *on* campus. Reggie still feels a close affinity to Sherman College. He feels more confident in Sherman's future despite being under the CCE's control than he did with Palmer and the other schools in 1975. The reason is that straight chiropractic has been defined by its objective now. That is the ruler by which Sherman will be measuring itself. In 1975, objective straight chiropractic was yet to be fully developed and traditional chiropractic, that practiced by the straight schools, was so ill defined that "procedures preparatory to and complimentary to" and diagnosis could be justified. B.J. defined chiropractic. It was not that his definition was wrong, it just left chiropractic open to so much distortion. Reggie tightened that definition so nothing is left up to the individual if he still wants to call it straight chiropractic.

Sherman alone represents Reggie's strengthening of the chiropractic definition and for that reason he has strong feelings for the school. Further, Sherman College has accepted him more than any other group. For many years he was persona-non grata on many campuses including his alma mater, Palmer College. Reggie wanted a place where he could call home, where he could speak to hundreds of chiropractors and share his vision. Spinology did not seem like it would ever afford him that opportunity. Straight chiropractic in general and Sherman College in particular, offered him a place and a platform to do what he so capably had done for many years, talk straight chiropractic. Thom Gelardi and Sherman College still have strong feelings for Reg. He has done a great deal to help Sherman and will continue to support the school. Reggie, for all he has done for the profession, has received very little recognition, even in the straight chiropractic community. He has definitely given far more than he has received and he would be honored and thrilled to see some sort of permanent recognition. Reggie is still searching for acceptance as he was when he was a teenager in the military. He truly wants to be accepted by the profession, at least one segment of it. He has worked hard to gain that acceptance in the only way he could, by stretching people's vision, imagination and perception and challenging their thinking. That type of individual always makes us better people but rarely receives our proper thanks and recognition. Sherman College is the only place that could possibly provide that recognition.

Reggie believes the purpose of his life is to make a difference. How much a difference is not something he can totally control, but he must make a difference. "If you don't try to make a difference, what is your purpose in living? ...Making a difference gives meaning to your life." Everybody should make a difference in their own unique way, according to Reg, that is the purpose of life and as he has so often said if you use anything for a purpose other than what it was intended for, you will ruin it. Whether it is using a Cadillac to plow a field, or a razor blade to sharpen pencils or a life for anything other than making a difference, it will be ruined. He believes chiropractic has and continues to be the best vehicle in his life to make that difference in the world. He says, "There is nothing in life that I could dedicate myself to, to the degree that I can dedicate myself to chiropractic." He has felt that way since he first heard the philosophy in Dr. Peruso's office and he continues to feel that way. On a Tuesday, he returned from a seminar on the West Coast. The next day he got a call from a student asking if he could speak at a California chiropractic college on Thursday, so the following day he was on a plane back out to the coast to do a one-hour talk to a group of students at his own expense. What's more, he was thrilled and honored to do it. At an age where most people, chiropractors included, are looking to slow down (or already have) Reggie is going at full tilt and plans to continue. In fact, he says that as he gets older he has a desire to work harder and harder. The older one gets, the less time you have left on this earth to make that difference so the harder you have to work to insure that difference is made. That is an entirely different philosophy from that of the world in general, who live to retire at age sixty-five and the chiropractors who want to retire earlier, often only working three days a week to begin with.

What continues to motivate a man after almost forty years to do that? Reg himself best sums it up in a 1996 interview with me,

> "Chiropractic is my life... I didn't even know if I had a philosophy before chiropractic. That's why I love chiropractic so much. It gave me a life, it put things together for me. It took me out of what would have been a drab, uninteresting existence making nothing but money into something that gives me a reason to be around ... If I did have a philosophy, I wasn't aware of it. Chiropractic crystallized it for me."

Reggie enjoys life. He wants to experience every aspect of it that he can. To drain out of it every drop he can. He doesn't take the time to regret anything. That approach to life has caused some conflicts with people. When he came back to chiropractic from Spinology, some thought he should return with hat in hand, apologetic and contrite for his leaving the straight chiropractic community. That was not even a consideration to Reg. What was done, was done, it was now time to move on to the next adventure in life.

Reginald Rafael Gold is a unique person with a set of unique abilities and skills, the most important of which is the ability to look at life and various aspects of it in a different way. He can take a concept, simplify it, make it logical and then present it in an articulate and lofty manner.

His gift to chiropractic began in Spring Valley where he started changing lives by changing people's thinking. On those Saturday nights where a hundred or more chiropractors and spouses showed up, Reggie shared and asked nothing in return except, as Dick Plummer says, "To bring a box of donuts." Reggie has continued to give to the profession. Most importantly, he has given to us a way of constantly looking for more in chiropractic without making it less. He has taught us how to change the philosophy without diminishing the heritage that the Palmers gave us, to expand our philosophy and simplify our practice to simplify our message and thereby expand its application to mankind.

Chiropractic will never be the same because of Reggie and what he has brought to chiropractic. He has truly made a difference. He has united the chiropractors on an objective and as a result, clearly and unquestionably divided the profession. He has given us a pride in chiropractic but at the same time humbled us with the philosophy. In recent years, he has shown us how to give more by becoming less. The enigma and the contrasts that are the man have clarified and simplified chiropractic for chiropractors, students and the public. For this, thousands of people are eternally grateful and countless others who may never even know his name will receive the benefits of chiropractic. Reggie Gold has explained chiropractic eloquently, he has been one of the seminal thinkers in the profession and he has done it with consistency for almost forty years. What Reg has said, thought and done will truly, in the words of B.J., "affect the lives of millions tomorrow."

APPENDIX

THE TRIUNE OF LIFE

This is Reggie's thesis for his Ph.C. in chiropractic. It is his most well known written presentation of the chiropractic philosophy, printed with the permission of the author.

INTRODUCTION

In the study of any philosophy it is necessary to examine not only the individual segments of that philosophy but also the effect of each segment upon the next. The philosophy can have meaning only if studied as a cohesive whole. Parts taken out of context tend either to confuse the issues and present distortions, or, at best, to permit only limited understanding.

Every once in awhile, however, a segment can be found, which standing alone, appears so complete in and of itself, as to be both a statement of the entire philosophy and an explanation of it. It can be understood without reference to the other segments, and yet acts to give those segments meaning and depth. It is, in fact, the crux of the entire philosophy.

If chiropractic philosophy can be said to have any such self-sustaining segment, that part must be the "Triune of Life." It, and it alone, can be sequestered from the whole and yet remain a totality within itself. It is at once a simple statement of the essence of the philosophy and at the same time, an explanation without which the remainder would have no reality. Failure to understand the "Triune of Life" must inevitably result in failure to understand the entire philosophy of which it is a cornerstone. The student finds himself confronted with a maze of apparently unrelated facts, meaningless hypotheses and bewildering paradoxes.

As soon as the Triune is understood, the paradoxes are resolved, the hypotheses take on meaning and the facts become cohesive. Thus, from disrelationship emerges cohesion, from complexity, simplicity and from confusion, clarity.

This "Triune of Life" then, should be an area of concentrated study, for it embodies the heart and soul of Chiropractic philosophy.
Making the Message Simple 227

The art and science of chiropractic while inseparable from the philosophy, necessarily confine themselves to the human body. The philosophy of chiropractic on the other hand is much broader in scope. It deals not only with the body or material substance, but also immaterial factors.

The "Triune of Life" explains the relationship between the material and the immaterial, and more particularly the link uniting them. These, in fact, are the three components of the Triune: Intelligence, Matter and Force.

In this thesis, Intelligence, Matter and Force will be examined in considerable detail. Each will be studied individually and in relationship to each of the others. The Triune will be dissected, studied and reassembled to show the purpose and function of each part and the philosophical significance of the integrated whole. From the study of this vital phase of chiropractic philosophy certain conclusions will be drawn by the process of deductive reasoning. These conclusions will then be offered as axioms, for the purpose of gaining a measure of understanding of the chiropractic principle.

Perhaps, at this time, a slight digression is in order to see why chiropractic prefers deductive to inductive reasoning. The word "deduce" means to "derive by logic" (Webster). Deductive reasoning is the process of studying known facts and self-evident truths and from them arriving at inescapable conclusions which are then presented as axioms. Deduction goes from the general to the specific. After study of the general has led to logical axioms, specific areas are examined in the light of those axioms.

Inductive reasoning proceeds on an entirely different basis. Induction is the study of specific individual parts and from them draws conclusions about the whole. It assumes that what is true of any part is necessarily true for all parts and for the sum of the parts. It also assumes that what is true at one time for one set of circumstances remains true even when the circumstances change.

Chiropractic is based upon a major philosophical premise. The major premise is the starting point from which all deductions are made. All conclusions are drawn from fact number one.

Fact number one, the major premise of chiropractic is that there is a Universal Intelligence in all matter constantly giving to it all of its properties and activities, thus maintaining it in existence. If this is a truth, it explains many things which bewilder the mechanistic mind. To use this premise as the cornerstone for an entire philosophical concept however, its validity must be demonstrated.

Proof is an eternal thing. In fact, proof can exist only in its own acceptance. It is possible, for example, to deduce from seeing that the ground is wet, that it has been raining. To prove that fact to someone who refuses to look outside is impossible. So it is with any proof. In order to constitute proof, the argument and evidence presented must first be accepted. Since acceptance is an individual act by an individual mind, this means, in essence, that one can only prove something to oneself. Nothing can ever be proven to another person. He can be shown logic and if it makes sense to him he has, in effect, proven it to himself. Any proof can be rejected by the simple expedient of refusing to use any of the five senses, or having used them, refusing to accept as logical the deductions thereof.

The presentation of a philosophical thesis is, in effect, an attempt to show to others the logic of one's own arguments and to have hat logic accepted. To try and inject one's philosophy into a closed mind is a hopelessly frustrating experience. Therefore this exposition will devote itself to a simple presentation of evidence in the hope that the conclusions are inescapable.

While it is essential to prove a philosophy or premise to oneself before accepting it, general acceptance by others is irrelevant. A philosophy does not become valid when a great number of people accept it. Nor does it become invalid just because a great number of people reject it. Its validity can only be measured in terms of its acceptability in the mind and reason of one individual person.

In considering the validity of the "Triune of Life" it is well to remember that not only is proof a very tenuous thing, but proof of intangibles is infinitely more tenuous than proof of tangibles. Since two thirds of the Triune are intangible and only one third tangible, the task is an imposing one.

I. UNIVERSAL INTELLIGENCE

Every good dictionary offers some half-dozen or more different definitions of the word "intelligence." Modem usage tends to equate intelligence with the power or ability to reason. Older and more stable usage suggest the "power of the infinite mind" (Webster). Perhaps rather than define the word, it would be better to understand its function. As in studying the body, anatomy is a stepping stone to the study of physiology; the mechanical being important only because it serves the functional, so in etymology, the practical purpose of the word is prime.

The purpose of intelligence is to organize and maintain organization. Organization is the prime manifestation of intelligence and intelligence the sole cause of organization. The two are totally interdependent. Thus, if the presence of intelligence is to be proven it is necessary only to demonstrate what may be called "active organization." Active to prove presence and organization to prove intelligence.

The major premise of Chiropractic states: "There is a Universal Intelligence which is in all matter, constantly giving to it all of its properties and activities, thus maintaining it in existence."

Since all of Chiropractic philosophy is based upon this vitalistic viewpoint, to accept the philosophy it is essential to accept the premise. Conversely, acceptance of the premise makes full acceptance of the philosophy a simple progression of logic.

Bearing in mind that proof exists only in recognition of the facts and logic presented, and that proof of an intangible is infinitely more tenuous than proof of matter, it merely remains to present evidence of the major premise in a logical sequence. Those who endorse the premise do so because they prove it to themselves by concurring with the validity of its logic.

To study the Universe as a whole is a task obviously beyond the scope of a finite human mind. The finite or limited can not comprehend the infinite or unlimited. It is impossible for the human mind to even visualize limitless time or limited space. Of necessity therefore the study must be made, and the evidence presented from some small and reasonable comprehensive portion of the whole.

Perhaps the smallest and least complex particle of matter is a good starting point. Let the atom, then, be the first object of study and see if it does not prove the existence of organization and, thereby, the existence of intelligence.

The atom consists of a number of tiny units of electrical energy. In its nucleus there are positively charged units called protons and a number of neutrons which carry no charge. Electrons, or negatively charged particles, maintain a constant and consistent pattern of orbit around the nucleus. The nature of the matter is determined by the number of particles present and the pattern or ring formation of the orbit.

Albert Einstein proved that matter and energy are one. Matter exists as such only as long as the electrons are maintained in organized orbit. It is the organization or more specifically the intelligence which causes the organization, that maintains the matter in existence by uniting its component parts together in an electrical bond. These component parts are not matter but units of electrical energy. If the organization is ever disturbed, the cohesive force is lost and the units separate with tremendous force as pure energy. It is only by organization of the electrical units that all of the matter in the universe is prevented from becoming one gigantic atomic explosion. Organization, then, is essential to the very existence of matter. Without it matter would not be and the universe, as we know it, would disintegrate.

Organization, however, is an effect and therefore must have a cause, It has already been shown that organization is always a manifestation of intelligent action. Universal intelligence is the cause of the organized state of the universe. It is, therefore, the cause of all matter. It is accurate, then, to state that all matter is created and maintained in existence by the organizing activity of Universal Intelligence. This is a rephrasing of the major premise of Chiropractic.

On a larger scale, a study of any of the myriad examples of nature shows a delicate balance in the harmonious inter-relationship of component parts. This harmonious balance is further evidence of an organization so vast and complex as to stagger the imagination. If ever any part of the balance of nature is disturbed, the entire structure is weakened. History is rife with examples of man's attempting to alter nature to suit himself. Each time, he has paid the penalty. He attempted to destroy the coyote because it attacked his poultry only to find that field rodents, which are the natural prey of coyotes, multiplied excessively. Without their natural enemy to keep their numbers in check, they over-ran the countryside, destroying thousands of bushels of cops annually. Finally man had to import and release coyotes to restore the balance he had destroyed. Similarly, in an attempt to destroy bacteria, man is breaking down a vital component of the nitrogen cycle by which saprophytes convert organic wastes into the inorganic state for utilization by plant life. If he ever succeeds in destroying all bacteria, he will destroy all life.

So it is throughout nature. A series of checks and balances exists maintaining the ultimate perfection of coordinated harmony. This harmony must be either the result of organization by a Universal Intelligence, or a random and undisciplined series of coincidences. No third explanation is possible.

Coincidences do, of course, occur. To deny their possibility would be ridiculous. But, for innumerable trillions of coincidences to accidentally coordinate-ordinate and combine to maintain the universe in balanced harmonious perfection, is a little too much for the logical to assume that such delicate equilibrium is the result of accident rather than intelligent organization.

No one would think of looking at DaVinci's "The Last Supper" and denying that its artist ever existed, or of hearing a Beethoven symphony and suggesting it composed itself by accident. How then, by any stretch of the imagination, can one listen to the symphonic harmony of the universe and deny its composer? How can one observe the balanced artistic beauty of nature and suppose that it happened by accident?

To deny organization in the Universe as a manifestation of Universal Intelligence, is to deny all logic and all reason and to fall back on insupportable superstition.

II. INNATE INTELLIGENCE

Since the topic under discussion is the Triune of Life, an effort must now be made to establish a relationship between Universal Intelligence and life. As has been shown, Universal Intelligence is that which maintains in existence all matter whether living or not.

It manifests itself through a series of universal laws which are immutable, and universal forces which are unswerving and without solicitude for the environment in which they work. One might well ask, then, how living things are able to survive through countless generations, when the very nature of universal forces is destructive towards structural matter. The answer, like the answers to so many vital questions, is basically simple. An understanding of it, however, is essential to an understanding of Chiropractic philosophy.

All matter may be divided into two great categories. Animate, or living things, and those which are inanimate or, have not life. Living things exhibit certain basic manifestations called the signs of life, which are:

1. Assimilation
2. Excretion
3. Adaptability
4. Growth
5. Reproduction

Inorganic matter, and organic matter which is no longer living, do not exhibit these signs.

It will be noted that each of the above is the result of organization and is, therefore, an effect of intelligent cause. This is why living things are called organisms and living matter organic. The words organ and organism indicate that the matter involved is "organized in a pattern of mutual interdependence." (Oxford)

The cardinal difference between the animate and the inanimate is the state of organization present. The inanimate is organized on a level no higher than the molecular. It is therefore maintained in existence but is incapable of manifesting any of the signs of life. It does not, for example, adapt to change in environment and, therefore, is at the mercy of the elements. Molecules of inanimate matter may become bonded together, by accident or design, to form masses with varying degrees of resistance, but as natural elements act upon them they are gradually broken down again to the molecular level. Each molecule exists as an independent entity without dependence upon any other.

Living matter, on the other hand, consists of molecules which are bonded together in an organized pattern. Each molecule exists, not as an independent unit, but as part of a coordinated unit.

The molecules serve definite purpose in the overall structure, united not by accident but by masterful design. All of the molecules present are organized for mutual interdependence with the various properties of each contributing to the biological integrity of the functioning whole.

When acted upon by the elements, all matter is broken down to the lowest level of its organization. Inanimate matter is reduced to molecules but not to atoms, because the atoms are organized into molecules. In living matter the molecules themselves are organized into cells, and the cells into tissues, and the tissues into organs and the organs into systems. Finally, all of the systems are united into the total organism or living thing. This total integration and inter-activity of all the molecules demonstrates the presence of a much higher degree of organization than in inanimate matter. It is this higher level of organization that permits adaptation to take place, with the individual properties of all molecules being selectively utilized for survival of the whole.

If animate matter has a higher degree of organization than inanimate matter, it necessarily follows that it also has a higher degree of intelligence. The more complex the organizational task, the greater the intelligence needed to accomplish it. There can be no denying that living things are more highly organized than non-living things. Therefore they must have some additional organizing intelligence.

It should be clearly understood, that reference is not being made here to the human mind. As far as is known, a blade of grass or an ameba have no ability to reason. Yet, the inter-function of their component parts is as intelligently organized as that of man, the most complex of nature's creatures. A tulip bulb planted upside-down produces a stem which curves one hundred and eighty degrees to pierce the surface of the ground and thrust upward towards the sunlight. This is intelligent action, neither random, nor haphazard, but a definite adaptive response to circumstances.

It is true that man is a reasoning creature, but that ability to reason is the product of a totally different type of intelligence. It is essential to differentiate between the two. It is to make the distinction between them, that chiropractic philosophy uses two different terms.

The power to reason and to decide upon a course of action in accordance with that reason, the ability to remember, the faculty to form value judgments, are all manifestations of an intelligence which man himself controls. This is called the Educated Mind; its quality and quantity vary greatly from person to person. It can be enhanced by learning or damaged by illness. It deals primarily with external matters.

The inborn wisdom of any living thing which maintains its parts in active organization for the purpose of function is called the Innate Intelligence. It is the intelligence responsible for all things internal, it makes the upper teeth grow downward and the lower teeth grow upward. It increases heart rate when we walk upstairs. It regulates the action of some two hundred and fifty different glands simultaneously. It maintains and coordinates dozens of organs, hundreds of muscles, billions of miles of blood vessels and countless trillions of cells. It never sleeps. It cannot be injured. It is as great in the moron as in the genius. It is always present one hundred per cent in every living thing, from the most complex, down to the simplest unicellular particle of life.

It is this Innate Intelligence which forms one of the three facets of the "Triune of Life." It could be defined as: "That part of Universal Intelligence which exists in all living things:. The specific localized intelligence by which living things assemble matter and adapt Universal Forces in a state of active organization."

Webster defines "life" as " the vital force, whether regarded as physical or spiritual, the presence of which distinguishes organic from inorganic matter." That which is living remains so by organized function. The Innate Intelligence is responsible for this organized function. There can be no life without it. It is the Life Force, the cause of all living function.

Although the presence of Innate Intelligence is actual and demonstrable, its location has to be theoretical. The brain is the organ through which coordination is maintained. All motor and trophic impulses originate there, and all sensory impulses are interpreted there. It seems reasonable to assume, therefore, that the brain is the place in which Innate Intelligence is located. In actuality, however, there can be no specific location for Innate Intelligence. Being immaterial, it does not occupy space. To say that it is located in the brain would be to deny that it is located anywhere else. Paradoxically, it is everywhere yet has no location at all.

The human mind, being finite, is unable to comprehend the infinite. Yet such is the nature of man's quest for knowledge, that he tries to understand that which is beyond his comprehension. In so doing, he necessarily distorts it by bringing it down to the confined limits of his imagination. He tends to visualize Innate Intelligence as some anthropomorphic figure sitting up in the brain, pulling wires, pressing buttons and giving orders to all body parts by means of a complete telephone system. It is this type of distortion of truth that causes much misunderstanding of Chiropractic, and is no doubt responsible, in part at least, for rejection of the entire philosophy by many lay people and Chiropractors alike. In actuality, they are reflecting not the philosophy, but their own distortion of it.

Acceptance demands either understanding or faith. Chiropractic is not a religion. It is not based on faith. It is a philosophy, and therefore its self-proof must be based upon understanding. To understand an intangible is admittedly difficult, yet the reality of dozens of intangibles is accepted by all schools of thought.

Electricity is an intangible. It is not directly observable by any of the five senses. Yet it is a very real thing, the presence of which is easily demonstrable by its manifestations. The same is true of the Educated Intelligence. Nobody has ever seen one, or heard it, or smelled or tasted or touched it. Yet nobody ever thought to question whether there is such a thing. By the very act of questioning, they would be using, and thereby, demonstrating there own Educated Intelligence. Innate Intelligence is similarly demonstrable by study of its manifestations. Could the perfection of inter-related harmonious function of the human body be random and coincidental? If not, the only alternative is that there is, inborn within that body, an organizing intelligence.

There is one major difference between the Educated Intelligence and the Innate Intelligence, and that is the quality of perfection.

Since it is a part of, and yet apart from Universal Intelligence, Innate Intelligence must be as perfect as the perfection of creativity itself. It is always 100% present and functioning 100% as the active organizing force of every living thing.

This characteristic of infallibility is an important one, for it means, in essence, that the body, by the wisdom within it, always knows what is best for perfect function. It further means that Innate Intelligence will always act in the best interest of the body at all times, limited only by the matter with which it has to work and the time available for such work. It is, in fact, the doctor of the body, with the great advantage over all other doctors of being right 100% of the time.

Hans Selye, M.D., in his great book "Stress of Life", records the findings of a lifetime dedicated to researching the dynamics of life. He states that life is a constant process of adaptation. Indeed, adaptation can be said to be the most significant of life's processes. This is not to suggest that other functions are insignificant or that life could go on without them. It means, rather, that all functions can be considered a form of adaptation.

The ability to change function instantly in response to need is a tangible demonstration of the difference between the living and the nonliving. A living body, when cut, moves instantly to initiate repair processes as well as the many other responses needed to adapt to the new situation. Every single change in internal or external environment demands a corresponding adaptive change by the living organism. Failure to make that change results in the same destructive effect on living matter that Universal Forces have on non-living matter.

Adaptation, to be totally effective, must be perfect, not only as to character, but also as to time. A change that does not occur at the specific moment of need does not fulfill its purpose. In fact, the net result of such a change may be destructive rather than constructive. Adaptation is a constant function of Innate Intelligence. Since the internal environment changes in thousands of ways every second of life, adaptive response must also be as constant and as rapid. By this method, and only by this method can the intelligence of the body fulfill its purpose of maintaining coordinated function, with each part doing its job for the benefit of the whole unit.

III. MATTER

Adaptation, then, is the expression of the organization of life. But, it is not life. Innate Intelligence alone is not life, but rather the intangible basis for life. The tangible basis for life is matter. The immaterial or intangible can no more be said to be life than can the matter or tangibles. Nobody would suggest that matter is life. It is an essential part of life but no more than that. The same is true of intelligence. Life itself is a composite of the two, consisting of the expression of one through the other. Life is defined by Chiropractic as, "the expression of intelligence through matter." Obviously, both must be present for life to exist.

It was shown earlier that all matter is maintained in existence only by the atomic organization by Universal Intelligence. All matter, therefore, expresses intelligence. If life is "the expression of intelligence through matter." then all matter has life in the broad sense, for it all expresses the intelligence that created and maintains it. A clarification must now be made to differentiate between this broad sense and the narrower meaning of popular usage. It is true that in the broad sense, all matter can be said to have life because it expresses the Intelligence of Creativity. It has also been shown, however, that the organizational state of that which we call living matter is at a much higher level. The difference lies at the level of organization and with the key word adaptability.

By popular usage, the word "life" connotes that which is not only maintained in existence by a Universal Intelligence, but is also responsive to an Innate Intelligence. The presence or absence of an Innate Intelligence is the determining factor of differentiation between the living and the non-living. The matter itself is structurally the same; the organization is different.

Matter is defined chemically as anything which has weight and occupies space. Any particle of matter can be divided and subdivided into smaller and smaller pieces until it finally reaches the state where any further subdivision would necessitate changing the basic electro-chemical structure of the substance. If that basic electro-chemical structure consists of a single atom, the substance is called element. If the basic unit consists of two or more dissimilar atoms, the substance is called a compound and the basic unit is a molecule.

Chemically speaking an organic compound is one containing atoms or carbon. In this thesis, however, the word "organic" refers to living matter or matter which has once been living. This represents no difference of opinion with accepted scientific thought, merely a reference to the fact that carbon-containing compounds are formed by a chemical reaction which takes place only in living matter. Every carbon-containing compound found in nature is, or was at one time, part of the cell structure of some form of animal or plant life.

When two or more dissimilar substances are bonded together physically, they form a mixture which can be broken down with comparative ease. When they are bonded together electro-chemically, they form compounds which can then be broken down only as the result of another electro-chemical reaction.

Compounds, then, are stable substances which can be formed or split only by chemical reaction. This perhaps gives some insight into one of the most interesting phenomena of the living body. The various glands and organs of the body function as complex chemical factories. Each one manufactures a multitude of different organic compounds for the body's use.

The newborn infant contains within it everything it will ever need throughout life with the exception of food and oxygen. As food is taken into the gastro-intestinal tract, it undergoes a series of chemical reactions. The first of these is analysis or breakdown of the compound into its component elements, which are then transported through the serous circulation to various glands and organs. Here they are selectively resynthesized into such compounds as the body needs. In this manner all body chemicals and all body tissues are made. That which was eaten for lunch yesterday is today walking, talking, flesh and blood. From a ham and cheese sandwich with lettuce and mayonnaise on rye bread and a glass of milk, the body manufactures bile, adrenaline, lymph, blood, eye tissue, liver tissue, brain tissue and all of the other multitude of complex body structures.

From dead, inert matter, living cells arise by application of the intelligence that is within. Obviously, in order for the glands and organs to function perfectly and to manufacture chemical compounds of correct quality and quantity, there must be an adequate intake of elements. This means that food intake must not only meet minimum requirements as to quantity, but also be of correct elemental quality or type.

The body is extremely economical in its use of matter. It wastes nothing which may be of value. Even that which is a toxic byproduct of some cellular function may be utilized as an essential substance by another cell in a distant part of the body. Normal muscle activity, for example, produces lactic acid which is toxic to the muscle cells and if allowed to accumulate, will cause tetanic spasm. Lactic acid, however, properly broken down and resynthesized, in a complex series of biochemical reactions, is a vital substance for heart physiology. When muscle activity increases, heart action also increases in order to supply more blood for the muscles. The extra muscle activity produces additional quantities of lactic acid which the extra heart action demands. Thus the laws of demand and supply maintain perfect reciprocal harmony within the living body.

After death, when chemical reactions in the body are governed only by unadapted universal laws, there is no such reciprocal harmony. Lactic acid accumulates in the muscles producing a total tetany known as rigor mortis.

In life, all of the matter of the body responds to the governing intelligence of that body, thereby, expressing or giving action to the intelligence. The body itself, of course, is composed entirely of matter. The matter or material substance of the body is the form through which Innate Intelligence expresses itself. It is the second constituent of the "Triune of Life."

IV. FORCE

In the foregoing paragraphs, the two vital constituents of the living body have been discussed. A body without intelligence would be a corpse. It would have no life. It would be unable to adapt to changes in environment and, therefore, could not survive. It would be inanimate clay. Matter without Innate Intelligence is not alive.

Similarly, Innate Intelligence without matter must be considered not alive. It would have no presence but, rather, would be an ethereal or spiritual manifestation without corporeal entity. There can be no life without matter.

From this, it might seem that life is the coincidental presence of matter and intelligence. However, the mere presence of both is not sufficient. Bacteria are alive and therefore indicate the presence of Intelligence. In a dead body there are bacteria. Therefore, in a dead body there is to be found both matter and intelligence existing coincidentally. But the body is still not alive. In order for there to be life, there must be matter and intelligence and a link to unite the two. Only in this way can matter express intelligence and intelligence be expressed through matter.

Life, it must be remembered, is not the presence of intelligence and matter, but the expression of intelligence through matter. Hence, intelligence plus matter still need a link to unite them for there to be life.

The link which unites the two is Force. Force completes the Triune and is just as essential as the other two factors. That which in Chiropractic is called "force", is called "energy" in the study of physics. The two are synonymous and interchangeable. There are two forms of energy. Potential energy, on the other hand, is energy which is tied up or stored.

The energy of force which unites Universal Intelligence with matter is potential. It is that which maintains atoms in existence, and also forms the electrical bond between atoms in a molecule. If a molecule is divided by chemical reaction, potential energy is released to become kinetic energy, usually in the form of heat.

The human body, like all other matter is composed of atoms and molecules and is, therefore, a storage house for potential energy. It is also a vast laboratory wherein chemical reactions are constantly taking place which convert potential energy into kinetic energy. The body is, in fact, a subsource of kinetic energy. It takes in potential energy in the form of food and converts it to kinetic energy by physiological chemistry.

All matter is the result of Universal Intelligence. Energy and matter are interchangeable by the formula $E=MC^2$. Therefore, all energy is the result of Universal Intelligence. Rephrased, this means Universal Intelligence is the sole source of force. This point is of particular importance because it gives some insight into the nature of force. Universal Intelligence is, by definition, perfection. Thus, that which it creates and maintains is perfect. All matter is perfect and all force is perfect.

Universal forces are the generalized forces of the universe. They are governed by Universal laws. They are absolutely not adapted to constructive purpose and will, therefore, act to destroy structural matter. They can, however, be adapted. The mission of Innate Intelligence is to adapt Universal forces for use in the body. The function of Innate Intelligence is to create forces to fulfill the mission.

The function of intelligence is to create force. The function of Innate Intelligence is to create innate force. Innate forces are adaptative. Their purpose is to adapt universal forces for the body's use.

A universal force may be beneficial or harmful to the body. Innate force is always beneficial. That is its purpose; its action upon universal forces is to change them to their exact opposite so that they work according to the laws of adaptation.

Innate forces are forces arranged by Innate Intelligence for use within the body. They are universal forces assembled or adapted for dynamic functional purposes to cause tissue cells to function or to offer resistance to environmental force. They may be used for adaptation of other universal forces which have not yet been adapted or to balance, annul, check, augment or otherwise adapt them, or adapt to them.

Resistive forces are those innate forces which are called into being to oppose the invasion of external forces into the body. They may be physical or chemical in nature, and are specific to resist a specific invasive force.

Invasive forces are universal forces which invade and act upon the body in an unadapted or destructive manner. They, too, may be physical or chemical in nature and call forth a specific response from innate forces.

When an external invasive force meets with an internal resistive force, the result is a concussion of forces which may be constructive and usable by the body or destructive and unusable by the body. When resistance is low the concussion tends to be more destructive.

The principle of a chiropractic adjustment is to intentionally introduce a specific limited external invasive force to the spine. This meets with the internal resistive force of the body and the resultant concussion of forces is used within the body by Innate Intelligence to correct subluxation. This is a classic example of force being used by intelligence to affect matter. It also shows clearly how external forces are adapted for use within the body. An incorrectly applied adjustic thrust would also meet with an internal resistive force, but in this case, the resultant concussion of forces would not be utilizable by Innate Intelligence and would either be neutralized to have no effect or would overcome innate resistance and have a destructive effect. An ill-timed or unbalanced resistive force may result in subluxations, luxations, sprains, torn tissue or fractures.

Such a mishap could occur, for example, by walking down five steps when only four exist, or by applying great strength to lift something thought to be heavy, when in reality it was very light. This would be using more resistive force than the occasion called for causing an unbalanced concussion. It will be noted that these unbalanced or improper resistive responses are always due to mistakes by the educated mind. Innate Intelligence being perfect, makes no mistakes. Only educated or imperfect minds can err.

To err is indeed human, and if man were "only human," as he so often claims in order to excuse his mistakes, he could not long survive. The mind that forgets to wind the alarm clock at night could not safely be entrusted with the trillions of regulatory tasks of running a human body. Universal Intelligence, therefore, assigns this task to a part of itself within each living thing and equips it with whatever forces are necessary to accomplish the job. These innate forces are the link between intelligence and matter and permit the intelligence to express through the matter. They are the third constituent of the "Triune of Life."

Mental forces are those innate forces which are generated in the brain and travel via nerves to all parts of the body. They are also called mental impulses and, incorrectly, nerve impulses. While it is true that they travel via neural pathways, they originate in the brain as an intangible result of mental processes and should, therefore, properly be called mental impulses. The rays of the sun are not called atmosphere rays just because they travel throughout the atmosphere. They originate from the sun and are named accordingly. So should it be with mental impulses or mental forces. Science has long sought to classify the nature of mental impulses, but since they are neither physical nor chemical, no answer has yet been found. The method of neural transmission of mental forces is described as an electro-chemical phenomenon and has been understood by neuro-physiologists for some time. But to understand their prime mode of transmission is not to understand the forces themselves. Recent experiments with "thought waves" at Duke University have shown that although nerves are a major pathway for transmission of mental forces, they are by no means the only pathway.

Chiropractic is deeply involved with the neural transmission of mental impulses, and more specifically with the interference to that transmission which is an integral part of subluxation. The innate forces generated within the body are always 100% since they are a result of a perfect intelligence. They can fail in their appointed mission only when their transmission is blocked. Even when they are overcome by excessive invasive forces it is not because of lack of perfection, but because of limitation of the adaptative powers of the body. They are still 100% perfect within those limits.

It was stated earlier that Universal Intelligence is the sole source of all force. That means that Universal Intelligence is the source of innate forces. Since Universal Intelligence is perfection, and each of its products and effects is similarly perfect, this means that innate forces are always perfect.

V. PERFECTION OF THE TRIUNE

By definition, everything in the universe, both tangible and intangible, is the result of Universal Intelligence. This means that all matter, all intelligence and all force are the result of Universal Intelligence. They are, therefore, all perfect for their purpose, 100% of the time. The only possible cause of imperfect action, then, is the superimposed influence of some secondary intelligence. That secondary intelligence is the human intellect or the Educated Mind with which man is endowed. Why man was given command of an intelligence which can result in imperfect action and the free will to decide when to use it, is a subject on which many philosophers have pondered and expounded. It is a subject too vast to be treated adequately as a side issue of this particular exposition, and no attempt to do so will be made.

Suffice it to note that all manifestations of Universal Intelligence are necessarily perfect. Thus, even the imperfections of educated mind must be perfect for their purpose.

Innate Intelligence is perfect, yet it cannot adapt to maintain the body in life if any vital organ is destroyed, or if two thirds of the body's blood is suddenly removed, or if nutritional or oxygen intake are cut off. Innate Intelligence has limitations of adaptability because the matter which expresses it has limitations of adaptability. Similarly innate force has its limitations of resistance and adaptability. When any of the aforementioned limitations are surpassed, it is not as a result of imperfection of any of the triune, but rather, a result of the perfection of the limitations granted to them and placed upon them by their creator. Universal laws govern all matter and all force. They are a prime manifestation of Universal Intelligence. They are immutable and inviolable. Man cannot intentionally or unintentionally break a Universal Law. If he acts contrary to a law, it will not be broken, he will.

The living triune, then, is perfect as to quality and quantity but has certain limitations within which it must work. Like all other effects of Universal Intelligence, it can exist only within the framework of Universal Laws.

Innate Intelligence is always 100% in living matter. It is perfect as to both quality and quantity in health and in dis-ease. It is either present 100% or absent 100%. This is the difference between life and death. There is no in between. Even in terminal illness, the intelligence is working at 100% perfection with whatever it has available right up to the moment of death.

Innate forces, being a product of Innate Intelligence, are similarly 100%. They may vary as to quality and quantity, but only at the dictates of Innate Intelligence. They are always 100% of what is needed at any body cell at any given moment. They do not lessen in dis-ease or impending death, though blockage of their transmission may render them ineffective.

Matter, then, is the only one of the triune which can be less than 100%. This pertains qualitatively as well as quantitatively.

The word "health" means "hale" or "whole." For a body to be healthy therefore, it must be whole. This is to say each of its components, tangible as well as intangible, must be present 100%. If a body is deprived of any part or parts through surgery, accidental trauma, pathology or congenital defect, it can never again experience total health. The Innate Intelligence , through its use of innate forces will utilize the parts that are left to the best possible economy for function as perfect as the imperfect matter will allow, but total health demands totality of matter.

Health, then, becomes a relative factor. Total health, having a prerequisite of total matter, must be irrevocably gone when a part or parts are permanently removed from the whole. This limitation of matter does not lessen the task of Innate Intelligence, because of a lessening of the matter through which it expresses. To the contrary, it increases the difficulty of adaptation and places greater stress than ever upon the remaining parts. Total health is then inevitably lost and all that remains is relative good health. That is to say, the best possible state of organized function under the circumstances.

It is said that a person is healthy when all of the component parts are working together in harmonious mutual function in response to a single control. If the matter is 100% then health can be 100%. If the matter is only 90% then the best that can be expected is 100% of harmonious interfunction of the 90%.

This is relative health. Ill-health or disease is the state wherein, regardless of the percentage of body parts present or absent, those that are present are lacking in mutual harmonious inter-function. 100% health is 100% organization of 100% of matter. Relative health is 100% organization of less than 100% of matter.

Dis-ease is less than 100% organization regardless of percentage of matter.

The word "function" means purpose. Since all matter, all intelligence and all force are manifestations of Universal Intelligence or Intelligent Creation, each must serve some intelligent purpose. That purpose is its function.

The function of intelligence is to create force.

The function of force is unite intelligence and matter.

The function of matter is to express force.

It can be seen from the above listed functions that life is a coordinated fulfillment of these functions. 100% of life or 100% health is the 100% co-ordinated fulfillment of these functions. In order for the functions to be co-ordinated, the principle of "time" is involved. The sixth principle of chiropractic philosophy states "there is no process which does not take time." This fact is so self-evident as to require no proof. However, to accept it as fact is not necessarily to recognize its importance. Adaptation, the very essence of the mission of Innate Intelligence is a process, and like all other processes, it takes time. Coordination takes time. Creation of innate forces takes time. Transmission of those forces through matter takes time, If the time factor is imperfect, either increased or decreased, the resultant function will be imperfect. If hydrochloric acid from the oxyntic cells of the stomach is produced too soon there is hyperchlorhydria prior to the moment of need. If it is produced too late there is hypochlorhydria at the moment of need. Perfect function demands perfect timing. The result of vertebral subluxation is to alter the time it takes to transmit mental impulses from brain to tissue cells. The result must be imperfect function.

It has been shown that of the three components of the triune, only matter can ever be at less than 100%. It would then appear to follow that the only cause of imperfect total function is deficiency of matter. This, however, is not true. It has also been shown that even when matter is deficient, relative health remains at 100% of its potential.

The concern of chiropractic is those cases where health is at less than 100% of its potential regardless of the amount of matter present. Chiropractic is concerned not with the degree of matter present but with the degree of expression of Innate Intelligence through that matter. Intelligence is always at 100%. Force is always at 100%. How, then can dis-ease or lack of expression occur?

Again, the answer is a simple one, yet is the basis for all chiropractic practice. The answer is that interference to transmission of Innate forces can and does occur. This and this alone is the cause of imperfect expression of dis-ease.

Obviously, whether or not innate forces can be interfered with, is a prime question. If they cannot, then there is no cause of dis-ease. Since there can be no effect without cause, this would mean that dis-ease could not exist.

VI. TRANSMISSION OF FORCE

Article 122 states:

"The cause of Dis-ease is interference with the transmission of mental impulse."

There is a tendency today to suppress or deny this flat statement of provable fact and to suggest subluxation, which is the physical representation of interference to transmission, is *A* cause rather than *THE* cause of dis-ease. This failure to understand the term "Dis-ease," and the equating of it with the medical term "disease."

The word "disease" implies an entity, a presence of something which has affected the body adversely. There are some 1,860 named diseases, as of this writing, each different and demanding different medical treatment. Dis-ease on the other hand denotes the absence of an entity. The entity that is absent is co-ordinated organized function, or relative health. Disease, or the identifiable presence of symptoms, can be manifested when the body is functioning perfectly. This takes place during retracing, and also during the repair process after the cause has been corrected but before repair is complete. During that time function is perfect for that body in its current state of unwholeness, but symptoms persist.

Conversely, dis-ease can be present when there is no disease. When subluxation is extant but before resultant tissue damage has reached the identifiable symptomatic stage, there is, of course, dis-ease or incoordination, but no disease. When Chiropractic states that interference with transmission is THE cause of dis-ease it refers specifically to dis-ease and not to disease.

Those who would state that a knife wound or other external trauma produce dis-ease, forget that all tissue present is still functioning at 100% of its potential unless, and until, interference to transmission occurs. Therefore while a wounded body may manifest symptoms or disease, there is no disease if transmission of innate forces is unimpaired.

Poisons on the other hand may produce both disease and dis-ease. The disease or symptomatic changes occur as a result of direct tissue damage (reduction of quality and quantity of matter). The Dis-ease occurs as a result of chemical interference to transmission. It must be remembered that the cause of dis-ease is not vertebral subluxation, but interference to the transmission of mental impulses. The art and science of Chiropractic deals with the location and correction of vertebral subluxations, and certainly vertebral subluxations are the most common cause of nerve interference. But nerve interference, and therefore disease, can be caused by other factors.

A severed nerve due to accident or surgery, nerve tissue destruction from a poison, intentional nerve blockage used in anesthesia and synaptic dysfunction caused by ingestion of aspirin or other drugs, are all possible causes of interference to transmission. Each of these by virtue of the interference, will result in dis-ease. Chiropractic, however, deals only with correction of vertebral subluxation and not with these other causes of dis-ease.

Dis-ease is incoordination or malfunction of that matter which is present and functionable, not lack of matter or lack of functionalbility of matter. It is true that 100% health demands 100% quality and quantity of matter. But less than that 100% quality or quantity of matter results not in dis-ease but merely in the body's having less to work with. The cause, the only cause, of dis-ease is interference with transmission of mental impulses between the brain or coordinating center and the tissue cells of the body.

Perhaps a study of force in general and interference in general, will lead to a better understanding of specific innate forces and specific interference of those forces.

The only source of force is Universal Intelligence. Universal forces are unadapted for constructive purposes. They are manifested in myriad ways. Food, drink, heat, weather, electricity and sunlight are examples of manifestations. They adapted, beneficial to it. Their transmission may be either direct, by radiation, or indirect, by conduction or convection via some form of matter.

They are always subject to some form of interference. Examples of such interference to universal forces are:

a tree blocking the sun's rays producing shade;
a rheostat reducing passage of electricity;
a grounded and shielded booth breaking a magnetic field.

Such examples could go on almost indefinitely. They are to be seen by the thousands every minute of the day and can be physical or chemical in origin.

It is significant to note that all universal forces, while able to travel by means of radiation, travel faster and more directly by conductive or convective means.

The bolt of lightning which "strikes" a house is merely taking the most effective mode of transmission. Telephone communication is less likely to "fade" than is radio communication. Electricity traveling via a copper wire is more likely to reach its destination at a usable strength than if radiated.

Furthermore, different forms of universal forces or energy exhibit a preference for different types of conductive materials. Due to the properties of the matter, some are better used to conduct various types of energy than are others. Water, for example, is a fine conductor for electricity but a very poor conductor of heat.

It is also significant to note that conducted or convected forces are more easily interfered with than are those which are radiated This is due to the confining nature of the conductor or convector. To block radio waves means that some will go around the blockage unless it too is extremely widespread. A lead shield to stop x-rays must be much bigger than the x-ray film or the bucky grid, because the waves spread in an ever-increasing cone from the points of emanation. Electric impulses when transmitted through air, similarly disperse, whereas, when they are transmitted through copper wire, they confine themselves mainly to that medium and do not spread.

In the living body, innate forces conform to the same laws that govern all other Universal Forces. They are transmissible by radiation as well as by conduction and convection.

They too are subject to interference by either chemical or physical means.

It has been shown that all matter is capable of conducting force or energy. Specifically, the innate force referred to as a "mental impulse" is transmissible by any type of body tissue. Cartilage having a high percentage of inert matrix in proportion to its living cellular structure is the body's worst conductor but is still a conductor. Bone is also a fairly poor conductor. Blood, muscle, tissue and particularly heart muscle, which is described as a neuro-muscular tissue, are high up on the list as efficient conductors. Nerve tissue, of course, being especially designed for the purpose of conducting mental impulses is the best conductor of all. It is the main mode of transmission of mental impulses, the physical means by which intelligence and matter are linked. It is also the place where interference to transmission takes place.

In order to understand how interference to transmission takes place, it is first necessary to understand more about the transmission itself.

Scientific research has evolved several theories of nerve impulse transmission. The most commonly accepted is that the transmission is electro-chemical. Each nerve fiber has as its outermost layer, a semi-permeable membrane which is positively charged on its inner surface. The permeability however is selective. That is to say the positive ions are able to pass through this hypothetical membrane while the negative ions remain on the other side. This results in a polarized state, or a difference in electrical potential between the two sides of the membrane (Helmoholtz's double layer). When the nerve is stimulated, there is, according to this theory, a physical and chemical change which results in an increase in the permeability of the protoplast. This allows a flow of ions in both directions and, in consequence the previously segregated ions commingle. This, of course, produces a point of depolarization at the point of stimulation. This depolarization creates a difference of potential between that point and the next adjacent point which has not yet been depolarized. This is called the action potential.

To be of value in transmitting the impulse along the course of the nerve, the depolarization and resultant action potential must be propagated through the nerve fiber to its destination. This is accomplished because the depolarization at the point of stimulation releases energy which is capable of acting as a stimulus for the next adjacent point. This new point then similarly depolarizes and releases energy to stimulate the next and so on. Thus, in the form of a wave, the action potential passes along the length of the fiber and constitutes the transmission of the nerve impulses.

Soon after the depolarization has taken place, constructive forces are set to work to restore the membrane to its original condition so that it is prepared to transmit the next impulse as and when needed.

In the event of a vertebral subluxation, interference to transmission occurs. This fact is demonstrable by means of the electroencephaloneu-romentimpograph although the actual dynamics of the interference must remain theoretical until the phenomenon of transmission is fully understood. If the above theory of membrane depolarization is correct then a simple explanation of interference is as follows:

The vertebral subluxation being a small local sprain produces inflammation as does any lesion. Swelling or local edema always accompanies inflammation. The edema is an excess of extra-cellular fluid which, of necessity, changes the permeability of the plasma membrane. The excessive permeability permits an untimely interchange of the sodium and potassium ions, thereby, depolarizing the membrane and rendering it incapable or less capable of normal function depending upon the amount of damage dome.

It will also be noted that the improper depolarization from a subluxation has the same electo-chemical potential as does a proper functional depolarization. It, too, releases energy which affects the adjacent point in the fiber causing, thereby, the improper conduction of an impulse.

The foregoing is by no means the only acceptable theory of the physiology of vertebral subluxation. Certainly the effect of the lesion upon the hormonal production of the nerve cannot be ignored. Neither can the compression factor which must occur when body tissue, in an osteologically confined space, are compressed by reduction of the bony lumen of the foramen.

Interference to transmission of mental impulses can occur to the level of the nerve root where it passes through the intervertebral foramen, or at the level of the spinal cord itself. This latter type of interference, produced directly or indirectly by the subluxation, has far greater injury potential than does the former. Whereas injury at the nerve root level can directly affect only the limited number of nerve fibers of that root, injury at cord level can affect any of the billions of fibers which comprise that cord. This does not mean, however, that nerve root damage is even relatively unimportant. On the contrary, since every body cell is dependent upon the efficient function of all others, to deprive one of its proper nerve supply is to injure all.

It must further be remembered that interference can occur on the afferent as well as the efferent side of the safety pin cycle. If the brain is at any time deprived of knowledge of the circumstances of any of the body's parts, it cannot intelligently act to bring about adaptative changes.

For perfect function, the link between intelligence and matter must be 100% intact. If an impulse arrives a split second later than its proper time, it is an improper impulse for that moment. Thus if a subluxation does not completely stop the passage of a given impulse, but merely slows it down, or for that matter, speeds it up, it cannot fail to produce malfunction or dis-ease.

It is this transmission of force which is the prime, and , indeed, only, concern of Chiropractic. Medical practice concerns itself with matter. Christian Science and Ontology to name but two, concern themselves with intelligence. Chiropractic concerns itself with the link or communication between the two. It was to emphasize this that B.J. made his famous pun.

Christian Science - always mind - never matter.

Medical Science - always matter - never mind.

VII. HEALTH

Health is wholeness, or 100% expression of intelligence through matter. When the "Triune of Life" is perfect, health is perfect. When intelligence, which is always 100%, is unable to express 100%, it is because force, the link, is interfered with or unable to be properly transmitted. It can also be stated that health is harmony; the maximum state or organization in which every cell is harmoniously functioning to fulfill its purpose for the benefit of the entire organism. It is a state of supreme order.

Dis-ease is nothing more nor less than a lack of organization or order. Thus, malfunction is dis-order. There is no such thing as a stomach disorder or a blood disorder, because the stomach and the blood have but one purpose: the total being. The total being is either in orderly organized harmony or in dis-ease.

Dis-ease, dis-harmony or dis-order are all one and the same thing. They are but a functional manifestation of a single fact. The triune has been violated. The intelligence is unable to express 100% through the matter because the link between them, the vital force, has been interrupted. Unless and until the triune is restored to its natural perfection, life must of necessity be diminished. This is the principle of chiropractic.

Federation of Straight Chiropractic Organizations Constitution

This is part of the document that Reggie created during the summer of 1976. It was "ratified" by those in attendance at the meeting at the Clayton Hotel in Davenport in August of that year.

I. Name: The organization is called The Federation of Straight Chiropractic Organizations, also known by the initials F.S.C.O.

II. During the evolution of language, words tend to lose or change their original meanings thereby rendering them equivocal, and a source of confusion and misunderstanding. Such has been the case in chiropractic. Distortions of the meanings of the terms "chiropractor" and "chiropractic" have brought about the need for clarification. Hence, the terms "Straight Chiropractor" and Straight Chiropractic" are used in this document to describe what has already been defined as "chiropractor" and "chiropractic" in the writings of Daniel David Palmer, the discoverer of chiropractic and B.J. Palmer, the developer of chiropractic.

    The adoption of the clarifying adjective "straight" before the words is an intentional redundancy and in no way implies that the words chiropractor and chiropractic, without the adjective, could or should have any meaning except that originally placed upon them. The term "straight" is used herein only to indicate that true, undistorted definition. It is emphasized that straight chiropractic is the only thing that can properly be called chiropractic, all attempts to the contrary notwithstanding.

III. Purposes

A. To protect and promote the right of the public to receive straight chiropractic care according to the following definition and scope of practice, and to receive full and accurate information pertaining thereto.

1. Definition: Straight Chiropractic is a natural philosophy of life and health based upon recognition of the inherent ability of living organisms to repair and heal themselves, under the perfect direction of the Innate Intelligence of Life, in accordance with Universal Law; and the art and science of properly locating, analyzing, and adjusting vertebral subluxations for the restoration and maintenance of neural integrity, in accordance with the philosophy.

2. A vertebral subluxation is a condition in which a vertebra has lost its juxtaposition with the one above, the one below or both; to an extent less than a luxation; occluding an opening; impinging a nerve; and interfering with normal transmission of mental impulses between the brain and the tissue cells of the body.

3. Scope of practice: The practice of Chiropractic includes:

   a. pre-and post-analysis of the spine to locate, identify and categorize vertebral subluxations, by means of Chiropractic spinographic x-ray study, Chiropractic instrumentation, Chiropractic palpation of the spine through its immediately adjacent tissues, and/or observation of structures related to the spine.

   b. the correction of vertebral subluxations by means of specific chiropractic adjustments.

   c. educating patients and the public at large to the philosophy and principles of straight Chiropractic.

   d. nothing else.

B. To promote the philosophy, science, and art of straight Chiropractic.

C. To maintain high ethical standards of practice.

D. To promote and aid in the development of high standards of professional competence.

E. To protect and preserve, by all legal means, the right of straight Chiropractors to practice their profession in all jurisdictions and to disseminate accurate information about it for the ultimate benefit of humanity.

F. To protect the integrity of the terms "straight Chiropractic" and "straight Chiropractor" as defined herein, and to expose for prosecution any practitioner of deliberately and dishonestly misuses them with intent to defraud the public.

G. To seek and work to maintain just and affective legislation, for the regulation of straight Chiropractic practice, as defined herein.

H. To support educational institutions committed to the principles of straight Chiropractic, as defined herein.

I. To serve as a central, national unifying body for any straight chiropractic organization (professional, education, layman or other) which is committed to the same principles, and to promote fellowship, unity, and cooperation among them.

J. To protect and preserve the rights and freedoms of its member organizations.

K. To raise and disburse funds to achieve its aims.

L. To employ salaried and unsalaried staff to perform necessary duties.

IV. Executive Officers

A. The Executive Officers are : President
Vice-Presidents (s)
Secretary
Treasurer
Chairperson of the Board

V. House of Delegates

A. The House of Delegates consists of a representative or a specified number of representatives from each federated organization, apportioned according to the procedures set forth in the By-Laws.

VI. Amendments

A. This constitution cannot be amended.

Consumer Rights in Chiropractic

The first of four essays from the "Excerpts From the Proceedings of the 1978 World Congress on the Future of Straight Chiropractic"

A health care profession has a moral as well as a legal responsibility to recognize and be responsive to the rights of the consumer. Chiropractic is no exception to this rule. Indeed, because of its humanitarian history and development, chiropractic should assume a position of leadership in this matter.

The nature and extent of the rights of the consumer can be discussed in six major areas of consideration:

I. Safety
II. Competence
III. Freedom of Choice
IV. The Right to Know
V. Fair Costs and Fees
VI. Education

I. Safety

No system of health care can offer benefits to every human being. Chiropractic, for example, can not help the unsubluxated. But whether we can help or not, we certainly must not injure. A famous adage attributed to Flippocrates translates into "First, do not harm." This applies as fully to chiropractic as it does to medicine.

The patient has the RIGHT, not the privilege, but the absolute

RIGHT to the assurance that chiropractic practice will routinely include the use of every reasonable safety precaution. The word “reasonable” is obviously one of personal and professional judgment, but because the life and health of the patient are paramount, and must never be jeopardized, any error must occur on the side of over-caution rather than under-caution, even at the expense of the right to low cost care.

A. Safety in Technic

A great variety of effective and valid chiropractic technics exist. The selection of which is to be used in any particular case is a matter of individual professional judgment by the chiropractor based upon the following principles:

1. The least amount of force which will accomplish the adjustment is the greatest amount of force to be used.

2. The amount of force can be reduced in direct proportion to increasing accuracy of both “point-of-contact” and “line-of-drive.”

3. Specificity, because it limits force to a particular pre-selected area, is always desirable.

4. Because chiropractic is based upon the philosophy of allowing the inherent repair mechanism of the body to function properly from “above down” and from “within outward,” the chiropractic objective is always to adjust as few segments as possible, and as seldom as possible consistent with the correction of the vertebral subluxations.

B. Case History

The meticulous and highly specialized use of a case history in chiropractic is a very important safety factor.

The history should elicit and record any and all information which could help determine the technic of choice or contra-indicate any or all technics.

All historical data which could contribute to residual weakness must be considered whether recent or long past. Particular attention must be directed to any history of falls, accidents or other physical injuries, surgeries, prolonged or serious illnesses and/or the prolonged use of drugs and medications.

Often consultation with family members (only with consent in the case of responsible adult patients) may be necessary to complete the history.

C. Physical Examination

Physical examination by a chiropractor can be divided into two categories:

1. That which is done to analyze the spine for purposes of determining whether an adjustment is needed, and if so, where and how.
2. That which is done to determine whether or not any technic of choice may be contra-indicated by the presence of physical factors.

N.B. AT NO TIME SHOULD A CHIROPRACTOR HOLD HIMSELF OR HERSELF OUT TO BE COMPETENT TO DETERMINE WHETHER OR NOT ANY PATIENT MAY BE IN NEED OF ANY THERAPEUTIC SERVICES.

The only purpose of chiropractic care is to locate, analyze and adjust any existing vertebral subluxations so that the body may better live up to its own inherent potential for life expression. Whether or not a disease is present, and whether or not a therapy may be desirable to treat any such disease, is irrelevant to the practice of chiropractic. Every human being under every circumstance, better expresses his or her life potential when no vertebral subluxations exist.

The only purpose of chiropractic is to locate, analyze, and adjust vertebral subluxations. For any chiropractor to hold himself or herself out to be competent in the areas of diagnosis and treatment of disease is an insult to the long hard years of training, internship, residency and experience which go into the making of a diagnostic physician. This constitutes the most blatant form of quackery and consumer fraud. Chiropractors are no more qualified to know when a person needs the services of a physician or surgeon, than a physician or a surgeon is to know when a person needs chiropractic care. There is absolutely no relationship between chiropractic and the diagnostic, therapeutic professions. The diagnostic therapeutic professions identify, treat, cure and prevent diseases. Chiropractic does not relate in any way to diseases.

D. Spinographic X-ray Study

Chiropractic spinographic x-ray usage bears no more relationship to the medical diagnostic x-ray than medical diagnostic x-ray does to the industrial x-ray. The same types of machine and the same physical principles are involved in all three, but there the similarity stops.

Chiropractic spinographic studies are not intended for, and are eminently unsuited to, diagnostic use. Their purpose is to furnish information relative to the selection of, and the safety of, the chiropractic procedures of choice.

1. Safety Factors

In the matter of safety, spinographic x-ray pictures proved information regarding such factors as increased or decreased bone density from that which would be considered average, and variations in structure, shape, size and formation of vertebrae. In addition, they supply information on paravertebral factors which may influence patient safety. Spinographic x-ray findings are considered in combination with chiropractic physical findings and case histories.

2. Analytical Findings

It must be clearly understood that a vertebral subluxation can not be seen on an x-ray picture. A vertebral subluxation has four component parts, only one of which deals with vertebral misalignment. Since chiropractic spinographic x-rays do not visualize even tangible nerve fibers, far less such intangible factors as mental impulses and the transmission or lack of transmission thereof, the analysis of vertebral subluxation must include other methods.

However, spinographic x-ray study does provide a certain amount of very valuable information to be used as part of the total analytical procedure, especially with regard to the shape, size and location of a particular vertebra, its physical relationships to adjacent structures and the planes of potential movement allowed by the configurations of articular surfaces.

3. Radiation Hazards and Safety Factors

   a. It is incumbent upon every chiropractor to be familiar with and utilize all factors and devices which will limit radiation to the absolute minimum and to the immediate area required for analytical and safety purposes.

   b. The taking of x-rays other than spinographics by a chiropractor can never be justified and constitutes a health hazard.

   c. All necessary procedures must be employed to ensure avoidance of radiation exposure to office staff, other patients and the public at large.

   d. To avoid any possibility of over-radiation, case histories must include prior exposure information.

   e. Re-x-raying must be restricted to only that usage which is essential for the continued safe chiropractic care of the patient.

E. Consultation and Judgment

While every effort must be made to incorporate chiropractic analysis and safety control into a science, it must be recognized that the actual practice of chiropractic is largely an art form and is primarily dependent on subjective judgment and upon manual skill and dexterity.

The seeking of a consulting chiropractic opinion, therefore, is highly recommended in all cases in which the chiropractor is in doubt as to whether or not to follow a certain course.

When, even after consultation, there is some question as to the safety of following any given procedure, the rule to be observed is "When in doubt, DON'T."

II. Competence

The consumer's right to competence in health care is so self-evident as to need no supportive testimony. "Res ipsa loquiteur." THE FACTS SPEAK FOR THEMSELVES. Yet when visiting a doctor of any kind, the patient must accept such competence totally upon faith. The diploma so neatly displayed upon the wall merely proves that the doctor graduated. There is no evidence as to whether he or she graduated first or fiftieth in a class of fifty.

The license to practice issued by the State merely proves that on a certain day, perhaps long ago, the doctor was able to satisfy a panel of political appointees, none of whom necessarily had any particular qualifications either as an examiner, or as an educator, that he or she could answer certain questions. The questions themselves may or may not have had relevance to the field of practice. Frequently, chiropractic candidates for licensure are examined exhaustively in such areas as biochemistry, microbiology, laboratory procedures, therapeutics, and above all, diagnosis, none of which have the slightest bearing upon the practice of chiropractic. The candidates are usually given little or no examination in subjects which determine competence in chiropractic matters.

It is obvious then, that neither the diploma on the wall nor the state license to practice offers the patient any great guarantee of a doctor's level of competence or even fitness to practice.

Until this situation is remedied legislatively by a revision of all licensing statues, the only protection of the patient's right to competence must come from:

A. Heavy emphasis in chiropractic educational institutions on philosophy as a means of developing both moral commitment and theoretical understanding in the students to complement their chiropractic arts and sciences.

B. Educational programs must be strongly directed toward developing skill, knowledge, and good judgment in the chiropractic arts. Any excursions into study of the subject matter of diagnostic/therapeutic arts are tangential and must not be allowed to detract from the teaching of the chiropractic arts.

C. Using annual conventions and any license renewal continuing education programs to reinforce philosophical commitments and to upgrade both physical skills and didactic knowledge in subjects directly pertinent to the practice of competent chiropractic, rather than to teach the arts and sciences of the therapeutic and diagnostic professions, as is the current practice.

Because the ultimate guarantee of competence lies only in the conscience of the practitioner, each chiropractor owes every patient a silent vow of honest service and integrity. This integrity necessarily includes the setting and maintaining of high standards of competence. Only when personal pride and acceptance of moral responsibility are strong enough motivation to overcome greed and laziness, can the public be truly safe from incompetence.

III. Freedom of Choice

The United States of America, being a Constitutional Republic, guarantees its citizens certain basic rights and freedoms. Important, though often overlooked among these, is the right to Freedom of Choice.

This right may not be spelled out in the first ten Amendments to the Constitution, but is nevertheless inherent within the spirit of the wording.

People have the right to choose to accept or reject any form of health care, provided such choice does not infringe upon the rights of others.

Perhaps of all of the constitutionally guaranteed rights, none has been so consistently violated as this one. The medical profession offers one approach to health. The approach considers disease as an entity which must be stopped, cured, or prevented if humanity is to survive and flourish. It is devoted to the principle and practice of diagnosis, treatment and prevention of diseases.

Because for generations this form of health care has predominated over all others to such an overwhelming extent that it was virtually the only one, there has been no choice. Absolute acceptance of this philosophy by government, industry and the private sector has led to its being viewed as synonymous with ALL health care. When government, industry or private citizens sought a viewpoint on health, the only one considered was the one based upon this approach.

There was no freedom of choice. Indeed, no real need for freedom existed because there was truly no choice. Only one philosophy existed. It is quite true that within this philosophy, there were considerable choices of method or school of thought, and there was freedom to choose among them. (The only limitations upon such freedom of choice were ignorance and fear of ridicule, if one chose a method not popularly accepted.) But there was still ONLY freedom of choice of METHOD rather than freedom to accept or reject the basic theory that diagnosing, treating and preventing diseases was the answer.

With the emergence and development of chiropractic philosophy, a whole new approach to health was uncovered. Instead of accepting the theory that diseases attacked healthy bodies and made them sick, chiropractic pointed out that healthy bodies resisted disease and that people who were unhealthy, sick, weak, or rundown were particularly susceptible to diseases. So the chiropractic profession devotes itself to correcting vertebral subluxations, not diagnosing, treating or preventing disease.

Vertebral subluxations are a significant factor in reducing the body's inherent defense and repair mechanisms. They reduce the body's ability to adapt to its ever-changing environment, and to otherwise express its life potential. The idea of chiropractic is to allow the body's own systems to function normally because health is held to be the normal condition. It is not the purpose of chiropractic to diagnose, treat or prevent disease. Chiropractic neither endorses nor condemns the diagnosis and treatment of disease. It does not offer advice or suggestion regarding diagnosis or treatment, nor the desirability of either. Chiropractic does not prevent disease. It does not relate to disease in any way. Chiropractic offers an approach to health different from diagnosis, treatment or prevention. Just as a well-nourished, well-rested body has a better, fuller, richer life on all levels than a malnourished, over tired one, so does a body free from vertebral subluxation express all of its potentials better than it could if subluxated.

The freedom of choice offered by the emergence of chiropractic philosophy is not one of "either/or." The fact that a person chooses to, or chooses not to, seek chiropractic care has no bearing whatsoever on whether or not he or she chooses to, or not to, seek good nutrition, get adequate rest, avoid poisons and pollutants or treat any diseases by any one or combination of the diagnostic therapeutic approaches.

IV. The Consumers' Right to Know

Concomitant with the right to freely choose must be an equal right to the information by which alone an intelligent choice can be made. Free and full access to pertinent information is an implicit prerequisite to freedom of choice. When information is denied, choice is necessarily obscured and thereby denied. Even a partial denial of information often leads to a total denial of choice. To offer the public freedom of choice while denying them full and complete disclosure of pertinent information, is to make a mockery of the freedom of choice.

The chiropractic profession must fully meet its responsibility to disclose to the public, all information relevant to chiropractic practice. It is not enough for chiropractors to fully and honestly answer all questions asked. They must recognize that many people have so little knowledge that they don't even know that they lack knowledge. It is up to the chiropractors, individually and as a profession, to take AFFIRMATIVE ACTION to fill the education gap.

Only by accepting full responsibility to educate, can chiropractic satisfy the patients' right to know or the concomitant right to choose.

A. Truth in Packaging

The first step must be for chiropractic to stop the deceptive practice of false labeling. The label "chiropractic" has a specific limited meaning. To apply that label to any other practice constitutes fraud just as surely does the practice of labeling as "ice cream" a product which fails to meet the federally adopted standards for such labeling.

The scope of practice of chiropractic consists of and is limited to:

1. Pre and post-analysis of the spine, to locate, identify and cat-

egorize vertebral subluxations for the purpose of selecting an appropriate adjustment procedure. The analysis may include chiropractic instrumentation, chiropractic spinographic x-ray study, chiropractic palpation of the spine through its immediately adjacent tissues, and/or observation of structures related to the spine.

2. The correcting of vertebral subluxations by means of specific chiropractic adjustments.
3. The educating of patients and the public at large, to the philosophy and principles of straight chiropractic.
4. Nothing else.

This represents the chiropractor's boundaries of expertise, and therefore the safe boundaries within which he or she is qualified to practice. Even when a chiropractor, by virtue of training and/or licensure, is qualified to practice various therapies, to do so would constitute fraudulent and deceptive labeling if the patient were allowed to believe that such practice was part of chiropractic.

Again, it is not enough merely to be qualified to give therapy, or to honestly and fully answer all the questions about it when asked. The onus in upon the purveyor to fully label the product in language understandable by the lay public. When the sign outside the door says "chiropractor" the patient must reasonably be expected to presume that everything that goes on inside, falls within the legitimate scope of the practice of chiropractic. If such is not the case, the onus falls squarely upon the chiropractor to make full and complete disclosure and to offer the patient freedom of INFORMED choice.

B. Truth in Advertising

"Truth in Packaging" deals with the topic of honest labeling. More, however, is required. The patient has a further right to know before submitting to the ministrations of any practitioner, the degree to which the practitioner is qualified in any or all of the various arts employed.

Chiropractors are trained in chiropractic. They are not trained to be nutritional therapists, physical therapists, acupuncturists, psychotherapists, or for that matter, any other kind of therapists. Whatever private instruction they may have picked up from reading or from discussions or from equipment salesmen, hardly qualifies them to practice such arts with any inspiring degree of competence. If in spite of this they wish to practice them upon any person, they have several obligations:

1. To explain that what they are doing is therapeutics and therefore not part of chiropractic. (This satisfies the "truth in packaging" requirement.)
2. To explain the degree of competence that they may or may not have at the therapy attempted based upon training, experience, etc.
3. To explain the dangers and contra-indications inherent within the therapy itself, even when competently practiced.

Any failure to fulfill these obligations would constitute a blatant disregard of human rights.

V. Fair Costs and Fees

Within the responsibility to supply information lies the responsibility to supply information about fees. For some reason yet unfathomed, the public seems reluctant to discuss money with doctors, lawyers and other professionals. This reluctance can and often does lead to serious, yet wholly avoidable problems.

Fee systems, whether simple or complicated, whether fixed or flexible, must be explained clearly to prospective patients BEFORE any service is performed.

Failure to do so creates unnecessary difficulties and violates the patient's right to freedom of informed choice.

Any practitioner is free to charge any fee he or she chooses provided full disclosure is made in advance, and provided there is no statement from which a patient could infer that any lesser fee would mean lesser competence.

Government and private insurance programs generally have a fixed schedule of fees. If a patient is accepted within the framework of any such program and yet is expected to pay privately in addition to what the program pays, agreement must be reached IN ADVANCE.

The establishing of "minimum fee schedules" by professional associations constitutes "price fixing" and is in violation of both the principle of free and fair competition of the marketplace, and of various anti-trust statutes. The patient is protected from exorbitantly high fees only by fair competition and is denied that protection by price-fixing.

VI. Education

Only by the establishment and maintenance of high standards of professional education, can the chiropractic profession live up to its obligation to be responsive to some very fundamental consumer rights. Inadequate or inappropriate education must lead to a serious health hazard to the consumer in a variety of ways.

A. Inadequate philosophical grounding would result in failure to understand the legal and moral boundaries of practice, and thus cause chiropractors to enter untrained or only partly trained, into other fields of practice.

B. Any inadequacy in the development of the analytical and adjusting skills that are the heart and soul of chiropractic practice must inevitably result in incompetent practitioners.

C. Any inadequacy in training in diagnosis, while not in and of itself a health hazard, becomes a health hazard if and when the practitioner, unaware of his or her inadequacies, attempts to practice diagnosis on a patient, or leads the public to believe that what is being done constitutes competent diagnosis. It must be remembered that chiropractors, by virtue of their training and education, are no more qualified to recognize the need for medical treatment, than medical doctors are to recognize the need for chiropractic care.

For all of the above reasons and many more, the establishment and maintenance of appropriate standards in the education of chiropractors is essential to the consumer's right to competent care. For the protection of the consumer, therefore, certain absolute principles must be observed in setting and maintaining appropriate standards for chiropractic education.

The guidelines for establishing criteria for chiropractic education must be based not only upon high academic standards, but also upon the RELEVANCE of the subject matter to the objectives of the program.

The prime objective of a chiropractic education program is to produce highly competent doctors of chiropractic who are fully qualified to safely and effectively deliver chiropractic care to the public.

No such program can possibly be undertaken until a clear definition and scope of practice has been established. For an education to be relevant to a profession, there must first be complete understanding and acceptance of what is to be contained within the boundaries of the profession.

The currently accepted four year program with its approximately 4400 to 4800 hours of schooling may well be longer than is necessary to produce a fully qualified straight chiropractor who will practice within the very limited scope and definition. At the same time it may be hopelessly inadequate to produce a chiropractic physician whose scope of practice closely resembles medical practice and differs only when such difference is mandated by law. Educational needs for one who seeks to be both CHIROPRACTOR and PHYSICIAN would naturally exceed the needs of either one alone. Just as one who seeks to practice forensic medicine requires an education in both law and medicine, so one who seeks to practice chiropractic medicine requires an education in both chiropractic and medicine.

On the other hand, trying to cram diagnostic and therapeutic subjects not pertinent to the practice of straight chiropractic into a four year program especially designed for chiropractors, means pushing aside relevant subjects to make room for the irrelevant ones. This results in a lessening of the time and effort that goes into chiropractic subjects and a consequent lowering of educational standards. To lower relevance is to automatically lower standards. The education of a chiropractor, therefore, must be both complete and relevant. In the matter of chiropractic practice, the chiropractor is the vendor, and the patient, as consumer, has certain consumer rights. In chiropractic education, it is the student chiropractor who is the consumer. The educational institution is the vendor who must guarantee the consumer rights of the student.

Chiropractic students as consumers have a right to competent and relevant education. They also have the same full rights as any other consumer, to receive from their vendor, freedom of choice based upon truth in packaging and truth in advertising. It is high time that all the professions and also the educational institutions which serve them become more responsive to the moral and legal rights of the consumers.

About the Author

Joseph B. Strauss, D.C., F.C.S.C., graduated from Columbia Institute of Chiropractic (now New York Chiropractic College) in 1967. Dr. Strauss was a professor at Pennsylvania College of Straight Chiropractic where he taught chiropractic philosophy from 1978 to 1994. He began writing for the chiropractic profession in 1991 with his first book, Chiropractic Philosophy, which continues to be read world-wide by chiropractors and chiropractic students alike. Dr. Strauss has written a total of 22 chiropractic textbooks.

In 1992 Dr. Strauss was elected a Fellow of the College of Straight Chiropractic. In 1999 he was honored as Chiropractor of the Year by Sherman College of Straight Chiropractic in Spartanburg, SC. Dr. Strauss has lectured throughout the United States and overseas in Japan, New Zealand, and England on the subject of chiropractic philosophy. He maintained an active practice in Levittown, Pennsylvania for over 45 years and is now retired from practice. He continues to write for the profession and offer his books and other products on his website ChiropracticOutsidetheBox.com. You can trust any of his products to be philosophically-sound, carrying the message of objective, non-therapeutic, straight chiropractic. Dr. Strauss also continues to speak at chiropractic seminars and conferences

Books Written by Joseph B. Strauss, D.C., F.C.S.C.

The Journey

Chiropractic Philosophy (3rd edition)

Toward a Better Understanding of Chiropractic Philosophy

Case Management for Straight Chiropractors

Practice Building for Straight Chiropractors

The Pivot Review: 1984-1991

The Pivot Review: 1992-1997

The Pivot Review: 1998-2003

Refined by Fire: the Evolution of Straight Chiropractic

Enhance Your Life Experience

Reggie: Making the Message Simple

Higher Ground

Still Higher Ground

The Green Book Commentaries (7 Volumes)

The Nature of Man

Conflicts of Philosophies

Chiropractic Philosophical Constructs

CPSIA information can be obtained
at www.ICGtesting.com
Printed in the USA
BVHW032100260921
617373BV00015B/1